CARDIAC

MW00635991

made
ridiculously
simple

Michael A. Chizner, MD, FACP, FACC, FAHA

Founder and former Chief Medical Director, The Heart Center of Excellence
Founding Director, Cardiology Fellowship Program
Broward Health
Fort Lauderdale, Florida

Clinical Professor of Medicine
University of Miami Miller School of Medicine
Miami, Florida

Clinical Professor of Medicine
University of Florida College of Medicine
Gainesville, Florida

Clinical Professor of Medicine
Dr. Kiran C. Patel College of Osteopathic Medicine at Nova Southeastern University
Fort Lauderdale, Florida

Clinical Professor of Integrated Medical Science
Charles E. Schmidt College of Medicine at Florida Atlantic University
Boca Raton, Florida

Clinical Professor of Medicine
Herbert Wertheim College of Medicine at Florida International University
Miami, Florida

Clinical Professor of Medicine
Barry University
Miami, Florida

Ryan E. Chizner, DO, FACC, MPH, RPVI

Interventional and Clinical Cardiologist
Cardiovascular Institute of Central Florida
Ocala, Florida

Clinical Assistant Professor of Medicine
Dr. Kiran C. Patel College of Osteopathic Medicine at Nova Southeastern University
Fort Lauderdale, Florida

Board Certified in Cardiology and Interventional Cardiology
Board Certified Registered Physician in Vascular Interpretation
Board Certified in Adult Echocardiography
Board Certified in Internal Medicine

Medmaster, Miami

ISBN #978-1-935660-35-4

Made in the United States of America

Published by
MedMaster, Inc.
P.O. Box 640028
Miami, FL 33164

Cover and artwork by Richard March

Dedication

To our family …
without whose love, support,
and encouragement,
this book would not have been possible.

About the Authors

Michael A. Chizner, MD, FACP, FACC, FAHA is a nationally renowned cardiologist and a Clinical Professor of Medicine at six universities in the state of Florida - the University of Miami, the University of Florida, Florida Atlantic University, Florida International University, Nova Southeastern University, and Barry University. He is the Founder and former Chief Medical Director of The Heart Center of Excellence and the Founding Director of the Cardiology Fellowship Program at Broward Health, one of the nation's largest public health care systems based in Fort Lauderdale, Florida. Dr. Chizner graduated with highest honors from Cornell University Medical College. He received his Internal Medicine residency training at the New York Hospital – Cornell Medical Center, and his Cardiology fellowship training with legendary cardiologist Dr. W. Proctor Harvey at Georgetown University, where he was the recipient of the Distinguished Alumnus Award. Dr. Chizner is Board Certified in Internal Medicine and Cardiology and is a Fellow of the American College of Physicians, the American College of Cardiology, and the American Heart Association. Dr. Chizner has served as Chairman of the Florida Board of Medicine. He has also served on the Editorial Advisory Boards of national cardiology journals and has been Director and Keynote Speaker at national and regional continuing medical education conferences. Dr. Chizner has written and edited numerous articles and books in cardiology. His best-selling book, *Clinical Cardiology Made Ridiculously Simple*, 5th edition, is currently being used in medical schools throughout the U.S. and abroad. Among the many awards and accolades he has received, Dr. Chizner has earned the distinction of being recognized by his peers as one of the top 1% of physicians in the nation in the first Top Doctor's List compiled by *U.S. News & World Report*, and has earned the honor of being selected as a recipient of the prestigious Marquis *Who's Who* Lifetime Achievement Award.

Ryan E. Chizner, DO, FACC, MPH, RPVI is a practicing clinical and interventional cardiologist, and an Assistant Clinical Professor of Medicine at Nova Southeastern University College of Osteopathic Medicine in Fort Lauderdale, Florida. Dr. Chizner graduated with a Bachelor of Science degree in Food Sciences and Human Nutrition from the University of Florida College of Agricultural and Life Sciences. He received his medical degree, along with his Master of Public Health degree, from Nova Southeastern University College of Osteopathic Medicine. Dr. Chizner completed his Internal Medicine residency training and General and Interventional Cardiology fellowship training at Palmetto General Hospital / Nova Southeastern University in Hialeah, Florida, where he earned the distinction of being selected to serve as both Chief Information

Technology Resident and Chief Interventional Cardiology Fellow. Dr. Chizner is quintuple Board Certified in Internal Medicine, Cardiology, Interventional Cardiology, Echocardiography, and Vascular Ultrasound. He is also board eligible in Nuclear Cardiology. Dr. Chizner has written numerous articles in cardiology published in peer-reviewed journals. He is actively involved in the education of medical students, residents, fellows, physicians, nursing students, nurses, and other healthcare professionals at all levels.

Acknowledgments

We would like to express our deep appreciation to Dr. Stephen Goldberg, President of MedMaster, Inc., for his invaluable assistance in the preparation of this book. Not only do we value his expert help and advice, but we especially appreciate his warm continuing friendship and support in this endeavor.

We are also indebted to Mr. Richard March, a uniquely talented illustrator and cartoonist, whose extraordinary artistic skills helped to enhance the text and pictorially "bring to life" our original concepts and ideas in such a delightful and charming way.

Special recognition and heartfelt thanks go to Ms. Stephanie Crossley, whose superb administrative skills, along with her meticulous attention to detail and ability to multitask, were essential to bringing this book to fruition.

We would also like to acknowledge and give special thanks to Mrs. Aniamma Geevarghese, APRN; Mrs. Kelly M. Roland, APRN, and Ms. Carly Yeckes, whose unrelenting enthusiasm, dedication, and faithful support were most helpful to the completion of the book.

Our heartfelt thanks extend to the many medical students, residents, fellows, physicians, nurses, and other health care professionals with whom we have had the pleasure and privilege to work. It is their passion for learning that continues to be an inspiration to us. This book has benefited greatly from their invaluable insights.

Last, but not least, we especially would like to express our gratitude and deep appreciation to our family – to Susan Chizner, Kevin Chizner, and Blair and Jonathan Steinberg – whose love, support, and encouragement helped to make this book a reality.

Michael A. Chizner
Ryan E. Chizner

Contents

Preface

Cardiac drugs are the cornerstone of modern cardiovascular therapeutics. The armamentarium of cardiac drugs used for the prevention and treatment of cardio-vascular disease continues to grow at an unprecedented rate. As a result, practicing clinicians and trainees often feel overwhelmed when trying to keep pace with the ever-increasing array of cardiac drugs available, and become frustrated when faced with the difficult decision of which drug to choose for which condition.

To address this challenge, *Cardiac Drugs Made Ridiculously Simple* is written to provide a lucid, straightforward summary of the current knowledge and appropriate use of cardiovascular drug therapy. Written by clinicians for clinicians, this practical therapeutic handbook distills basic clinical concepts to a concise, clear minimum, while including essential information on the latest pharmacologic treatment recommendations to help guide clinical decision making in the hospital or outpatient setting.

The book is organized into three parts. Part I presents the reader with an overall clinical perspective on modern cardiovascular therapy. The chapters in Part II focus on the most common cardiac drugs in cardiology, along with their mechanisms, clinical indications, and strategy of use. The chapters in Part III provide the reader with an up-to-date, "evidence-based" approach to the pharmacologic treatment of a broad spectrum of cardiac disease states and conditions encountered in clinical practice. Where appropriate, current indications for the latest cardiac surgical, device, and "catheter-based" interventional therapeutic techniques are also discussed.

In addition to the written text, the numerous figures, tables, flow charts, algorithms, and pearls, interspersed throughout the book, serve as a visual aid to make the learning and understanding of cardiovascular drug therapy easy, memorable, and enjoyable. A concise, yet comprehensive summary table of the most commonly used cardiac drugs, along with their clinical indications, dosages, and other pertinent facts is provided in the readily accessible, user-friendly Appendix. When more in-depth information is required, the reader is encouraged to refer to the companion text, *Clinical Cardiology Made Ridiculously Simple*, now in its fifth edition.

It is our sincere hope that the information provided in this book will be extremely useful for board exam preparation and course study, and will prove to be of great value to all clinicians and trainees who strive to provide the highest quality care to their patients with, or at risk for, cardiovascular disease.

We welcome your comments and suggestions for future editions.

Michael A. Chizner, MD
Ryan E. Chizner, DO

PART I.   CARDIOVASCULAR THERAPEUTICS

Therapeutic decision making in cardiology proceeds through an orderly sequence of events that begins with a careful clinical history and physical examination. Diagnostic laboratory tests are then performed, as needed, and the results integrated into an assessment of the probability of cardiac disease. Based on this information and the evidence to support various therapeutic interventions, appropriate treatment can begin. It is important to understand the natural history of the cardiac disease, both untreated and treated, before recommending drug, device or surgical interventions. Keep in mind that a disease encountered during an earlier stage may require less aggressive intervention than at a later stage in the natural history. Decisions regarding the appropriate treatment of the cardiac patient are based on the best scientific evidence available and guided by sound clinical judgment. This can be acquired only through clinical experience gleaned by caring for many patients over a long period of time. Remember, *good judgment comes from experience... which often comes from bad judgment.*

Chapter 1.   General Considerations and Treatment Goals

Before considering what may be life-long treatment for the patient, you should consider the long-term efficacy of the drug and/or procedure, and what negative effects can be expected (i.e., is the treatment worse than the disease?). The risk of treatment should be outweighed by its benefit to the patient. It is surprising how uncritical today's practitioners can be in embracing new therapies without asking critical questions regarding proof of efficacy. With new treatments being advertised to the lay public (through the Internet, television commercials, and other print media), and patients often requesting them before they can be properly evaluated, you should develop a healthy skepticism about claims regarding a new drug's efficacy and/or safety, and seek out objective sources before prescribing (**Fig. 1-1**). The history of cardiovascular therapeutics includes many examples of new treatments initially recommended enthusiastically, but later abandoned as

Figure 1-1

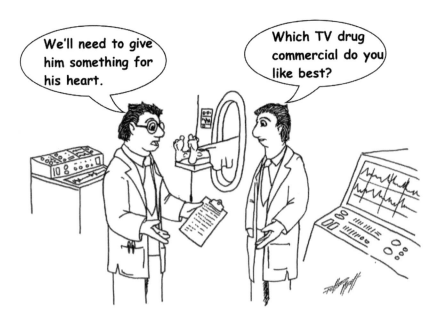

useless or worse, even harmful. Some of these new therapies were actually tested by well-designed clinical trials with results seemingly indicative of effectiveness, yet later disproved, and even taken off the market after discovery of serious side effects. You would do well to follow a conservative strategy of "watchful waiting" whenever possible, before pushing your patient too rapidly into new treatments. There are times, however, when a major "breakthrough" in management is demonstrated to be safe and effective and therefore should be utilized sooner.

The haphazard administration of a large number of drugs is more likely to create harm than benefit. Always keep in mind factors such as side effects, ease of administration, desires and/or compliance of the patient, and cost considerations when determining the appropriate therapy for the individual patient. Remember to take a "good look" at your patient. After all, you are not treating a disease, you are treating a patient who has the disease. Two patients with the same cardiac condition may respond differently to the same medication. What may be an effective medication for one patient may be toxic for another. Most drug side effects can be prevented by a careful review of the patient's clinical database (i.e., age, liver and kidney function, presence of associated diseases, and other medications). Adverse drug reactions are often dose-dependent, and correct dosing minimizes patient's risk.

In addition to compiling a list of medications and their side effects, specifically inquire about whether your patient is allergic to iodine, which is present in the contrast medium used during cardiac catheterization and computerized tomography (CT) scanning. Keep in mind that patients, who claim to have an aspirin allergy, but instead have had gastrointestinal (GI) upset, are usually able to tolerate aspirin after undergoing stent implantation.

Figure 1-2. Ask your patients (or their spouses) to describe how they take their medication. Safe and appropriate medication use requires close adherence to the five "*rights*": *right* patient, *right* drug, *right* dose, *right* route, *right* time.

It is important to find out what medicines, prescription or nonprescription (i.e., over-the-counter, including herbal remedies) the patient is taking and how they are being administered. Are they being swallowed, inhaled (e.g., bronchodilators, steroids) or applied topically (e.g., timolol eye drops)? Some cardiac medications may actually harm patients, and even increase their chances of dying. Sometimes cardiac medications can mimic the very signs and symptoms for which they were given! For example: class IA and III anti-arrhythmic agents used in the treatment of ventricular tachycardia (VT) can prolong the QT interval, and cause the VT called "*torsades de pointes*" and recurrent syncope, and thus, ironically produce the same fatal ventricular arrhythmia that one is trying to prevent.

Other causes of this potentially lethal ventricular arrhythmia include diuretics (due to hypokalemia, hypomagnesemia), phenothiazines, tricyclic antidepressants, liquid protein diets, and the use of certain non-sedating antihistamines, e.g., terfenadine (Seldane), astemizole (Hismanal) in combination with cytochrome P-450 inhibitors (e.g., erythromycin, and other macrolide antibiotics) and grapefruit juice. This is not merely "pulp fiction"! You should instruct your patients to refrain from drinking grapefruit juice when they are taking drugs that are known to be susceptible to this interaction.

3

Figure 1-2

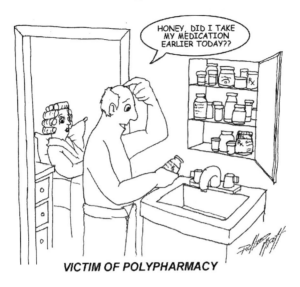

VICTIM OF POLYPHARMACY

Note: Patients are frequently victims of polypharmacy, and despite the best of intentions, often make inadvertent medication errors (especially the elderly).

A dry, nonproductive cough is a particularly annoying side effect of long-term angiotensin converting enzyme (ACE) inhibitor therapy. It occurs in ~5-20% of patients, and is thought to be caused by increased bradykinin levels. There is no relationship between the dose of the ACE inhibitor and the development of cough. Although cough most often occurs within the first few weeks of therapy, it may occur 6 months after the initiation of an ACE inhibitor. In patients with known congestive heart failure (CHF), the presence of chronic cough may also be a manifestation of suboptimal treatment. Keep in mind that a patient who has developed a cough from an ACE inhibitor in the past will not be pleased to find out that his or her "new" medication is another form of the offending agent. Switching to a different ACE inhibitor is rarely effective in reducing this bothersome side effect. Angiotensin receptor blockers (ARBs) are a better alternative for most patients with intractable cough.

Worthy of mention, antiarrhythmic drugs are not recommended for premature ventricular contractions (PVCs) in asymptomatic patients without cardiac disease. Instead, you should encourage your patient to avoid stimulants (e.g., nicotine, caffeine, alcohol). Keep in mind that hypokalemia and hypomagnesemia, which may occur in patients taking diuretics, can also precipitate PVCs, and should be corrected.

Figure 1-3 summarizes potential side effects (both cardiovascular and non-cardiovascular) that can arise from drugs currently utilized for the treatment of various heart conditions.

Figure 1-3

SYMPTOMS ATTRIBUTABLE TO CARDIOVASCULAR DRUGS*

SYMPTOM	CARDIOVASCULAR DRUG/MECHANISM
CNS	
Headache	Nitroglycerin
Syncope	Class IA and III antiarrhythmic agents
	(torsades de pointes) Beta blockers } bradycardia
	Diuretics, vasodilators (e.g., nitrates,
	calcium channel blockers, α-blockers),
	ACE inhibitors, hydralazine $\left.\vphantom{\begin{array}{c}1\\2\\3\end{array}}\right\}$ hypotension
	Warfarin—blood loss
Tremor, ataxia	Amiodarone
Tremor, confusion, stupor, coma, seizures	Lidocaine
Confusion, delirium, disorientation	Digitalis
Gastrointestinal	
Xerostomia	Disopyramide
Anorexia	Digitalis
Nausea, vomiting	Quinidine, digitalis
Diarrhea	Quinidine
Constipation	Verapamil, cholestyramine
Peptic disease	Nicotinic acid
Pulmonary	
Shortness of breath	Ticagrelor
Cough	ACE inhibitors, ticagrelor
Pulmonary fibrosis	Amiodarone
Genitourinary	
Nocturia	Diuretics
Hesitancy	Disopyramide
Impotence	Beta blockers
Renal insufficiency	ACE inhibitors, contrast medium
Endocrine	
Hyper/hypothyroid	Amiodarone
Diabetes aggravated	Nicotinic acid
Hypoglycemia masked	Beta blockers
Musculoskeletal	
Arthritis, lupus	Procainamide, hydralazine
Muscle weakness, cramps	Diuretics/electrolyte depletion
Muscle aches and pains (Myositis syndrome)	"Statins"
Cutaneous	
Sunlight sensitivity	Amiodarone
Flushing	Nicotinic acid
Fatigue/lethargy	Beta blockers
Gynecomastia	Digitalis, spironolactone

*Note: Most of the drugs used in cardiology have unwanted, and sometimes serious, side effects on the heart and other organs. These adverse effects must be carefully sought in all patients taking cardiac drugs.

Cardiac patients should be counseled regarding the risks of using drugs e.g., sildenafil (Viagra) to treat erectile dysfunction. Sildenafil is potentially hazardous in patients with acute coronary syndromes, CHF, borderline hypotension and low volume status, and complicated antihypertensive therapy since this agent is also a systemic vasodilator and it may exacerbate hypotension. Recent nitrate use is an absolute contraindication to use of Viagra-like agents (due to the potential for severe hypotension). In the management of acute coronary syndromes developing after sildenafil use, no nitrates should be administered within the first 24 hours (but other routine therapy should not be withheld). Also keep in mind that erectile dysfunction may be one of the side effects seen in patients taking certain cardiac medications (e.g., beta blockers and antihypertensive agents).

The goals of treatment in cardiology are to relieve symptoms, improve quality of life, slow disease progression, and prolong survival. Examples include:

- Restoration of normal sinus rhythm by chemical or electrical cardioversion
- Control of rapid ventricular response of atrial fibrillation and other supraventricular tachycardias (SVTs) by beta blockers, rate-slowing calcium channel blockers, digoxin, or catheter ablation
- Control of blood pressure by antihypertensive medication
- Reducing elevated blood cholesterol levels by "statins" and other lipid-reducing agents
- Prevent stroke and transient ischemic attack (TIA) in atrial fibrillation with warfarin or novel oral anticoagulants (NOACs)
- Restoration of coronary blood flow by thrombolytic therapy or direct percutaneous coronary intervention (PCI)
- Cure of infective endocarditis by antibiotics
- Correction of valvular stenosis and/or regurgitation by valve repair or replacement
- Treatment of CHF by ACE inhibitors, ARBs, angiotensin receptor neprilysin inhibitor, beta blockers, diuretics, and digoxin
- Relief of angina pectoris by nitrates, beta blockers, calcium channel blockers, PCI or coronary artery bypass graft (CABG) surgery
- Treatment of acute myocardial infarction (MI) by reperfusion therapy
- Treatment of syncope due to potentially life-threatening pauses or ventricular tachyarrhythmias by implantable pacemaker or implantable cardioverter-defibrillator (ICD)

It is not possible to manage heart disease as an isolated entity. Many patients with heart disease have other medical problems that may influence their condition adversely, and treatment of their cardiac problem may worsen other coexistent conditions. Furthermore, several cardiac drugs may manifest some form of interaction with each other or with noncardiac drugs. (**Figure 1-4**). For example, studies have implicated certain proton pump inhibitors (PPIs), particularly omeprazole (Prilosec), used concomitantly to decrease the risk of GI bleeding, as drugs that can interfere with hepatic cytochrome P450 2C19 enzymatic activation of clopidogrel (Plavix), and decrease its antiplatelet effect. Although some PPIs may interfere with platelet inhibition, there is no convincing evidence to date of an impact on clinical outcome. Nevertheless, it is vital for the practitioner to be aware of these interactions, which may be potentially harmful to patients.

Figure 1-4

DRUG-DRUG INTERACTIONS

COMMON DRUG INTERACTIONS	CLINICAL EFFECT
• Digoxin ± beta blocker ± non dihydro-pyridine calcium channel blocker (diltiazem, verapamil) ± amiodarone	Sinus bradycardia
• Nitrates ± diuretic ± vasodilator ± α-blocker ± calcium channel blocker	Postural hypotension
• ACE inhibitor ± spironolactone ± NSAID	Hyperkalemia
• Terfenadine, astemizole ± class I or III antiarrhythmic agent ± macrolide antibiotic ± grapefruit juice	Prolongation of QT interval and torsades de pointes
• Aspirin ± clopidogrel ± warfarin ± ginkgo biloba ± vitamin E	Increased bleeding
• ACE inhibitor ± diuretic ± NSAID	Azotemia
• Insulin ± oral hypoglycemic agent ± beta blocker	Hypoglycemic episode—prolonged or unrecognized (masking of hypoglycemic symptoms)
• Beta agonist ± theophylline ± anticholinergic agent	Aggravation of angina and/or arrhythmias
• Digoxin ± amiodarone ± quinidine ± verapamil ± propafenone	Increased serum digoxin levels and/or signs of digitalis toxicity
• Clopidogrel ± proton pump inhibitor (PPI)	PPI may decrease antiplatelet effect of clopidogrel

Chapter 2. Evidence-Based Medicine and Clinical Practice Guidelines

Over the past few decades, randomized clinical trial data, so-called *"evidence-based medicine,"* has emerged as an important tool to improve the quality of patient care. A large number of practice guidelines in cardiology are now available to assist the practitioner in clinical decision making. Good clinical judgment, however, is required to determine whether the guidance applies to the individual patient or if exceptions exist ("no one size fits all").

As in all of medicine, the goals of cardiovascular therapy, whether pharmacological, interventional, or surgical, must be clear in the practitioner's mind, and the patient should be educated as to the potential benefits and risks. If there is no anticipated mortality benefit, and the patient is not feeling ill, potentially risky treatment is not advisable. Keep in mind the dictum, *"primum non nocere"*, i.e., first, do no harm. In many cases, patient education and promotion of preventative measures, including a "heart healthy" diet; exercise; smoking cessation; BP, lipid, and glucose control; and weight reduction (if appropriate), ultimately may be the more effective therapy than treating the immediate problem. Remember, "an ounce of prevention is worth a pound of cure."

PART II. CARDIAC DRUGS AND THEIR USES

The introduction of new cardiac drugs and the new applications of standard drugs has resulted in significant changes in the clinical management of the patient with cardiovascular disease. The following chapters discuss the common cardiac drugs and their mechanisms. These drugs may have multiple uses for various cardiac conditions. Part III will focus on the common (and not so common) cardiac conditions encountered in clinical practice, and show how the drugs discussed in these chapters are used in those situations.

The different kinds of problems in cardiology require different pharmacologic treatment strategies:

- Acute and chronic coronary artery disease (CAD): Try to improve coronary artery blood flow through dilation of coronary arteries. Decrease myocardial oxygen demand through dilation of peripheral veins (preload reduction) and arteries (afterload reduction) and decreased myocardial contractility. Deal with acute and chronic thrombosis with thrombolytics, antiplatelet and antithrombotic agents and anticoagulants.

- Congestive heart failure (CHF) with problems of systolic or diastolic dysfunction:When there is systolic dysfunction, it may help to increase cardiac contractility and/or decrease peripheral resistance (e.g., lowering blood pressure) to make it easier to pump out the blood and increase cardiac output. With diastolic dysfunction, slowing the heart to allow more time for diastolic filling may be beneficial.

- Hypertension: Lower the blood pressure. Raise BP in significant hypotension.

- Dyslipidemia: Correct the lipid abnormality.

- Cardiac arrhythmias: Speed up a pathological bradycardia; slow a tachycardia; reduce the excitability of an ectopic focus in the atria, His-bundle system, or ventricles; decrease conduction along an aberrant pathway.

Advances in pharmacology, including combination medications (so-called "polypills"), have provided the practitioner with a wide array of effective cardiac drugs. Certain agents have become the "cornerstones" of modern cardiac therapy. These include:

- Beta blockers
- Calcium channel blockers

- Nitrates
- Angiotensin-converting enzyme (ACE) inhibitors
- Angiotensin receptor blockers (ARBs)
- Digitalis and other inotropic agents
- Diuretics
- Aspirin and other antiplatelet agents
- Thrombolytic agents and anticoagulants
- Lipid controlling drugs
- Antiarrhythmic agents

Chapter 3.   Beta Blockers

Drugs that act on the adrenergic receptors of the sympathetic nervous system have particular value in cardiology.

Figure 3-1. Location and effects of stimulation of adrenergic receptors. Beta-1 receptors are found on cardiac muscle cells, including the modified muscle cells of the SA and AV nodes, which are part of the pacemaker and conduction system of the heart. Stimulation of beta-1 receptors increases heart rate (by stimulating the Sinoatrial [SA] node), increases conduction velocity through the atrioventricular (AV) node, cardiac muscle contractility, and automaticity of the pacemakers, with a net increase in cardiac output. Stimulating these receptors (beta-1 agonists) may be of value to increase cardiac output, but blocking (beta-1 antagonists) may be of value when there is need to:

- Decrease the oxygen demand of the heart by decreasing heart rate and contractility
- Decrease a tachyarrhythmia by slowing conduction through the AV node and decreasing the automaticity of an abnormal ectopic pacemaker.

Beta-1 receptors are also found on granular cells in the kidney, where stimulation increases renin secretion. Renin initiates a chain reaction that results in the production of angiotensin II and aldosterone. Angiotensin II has powerful vasoconstrictive effects and aldosterone stimulates the renal tubules to reabsorb sodium (and, passively, water), thereby increasing blood pressure and blood volume (**Figure 6-1**). Increasing blood pressure may be useful in hypotensive states, but decreasing BP through beta-1 blockers may also be important, e.g. to reduce the stress (afterload) on cardiac contraction, or to treat hypertension.

Beta-2 receptors are found in the trachea and bronchioles and arterioles (but not in the skin or brain arterioles). Stimulating them will cause *vasodilation* and also dilation of the trachea and bronchioles. Thus, beta-2 blockers may aggravate coronary vasospasm, Raynaud's phenomenon, and intermittent claudication by inhibiting arteriolar vasodilation and leaving α-mediated vasoconstriction unopposed. They may also induce bronchospasm. It is therefore very important, when using a beta-blocker to understand whether it nonspecifically blocks both beta-1 and beta-2 receptors (and/or alpha receptors) or acts more specifically. In general, beta-1 specific blockers are preferred in cardiology.

Alpha-1 receptors reside on arterioles and veins. Stimulating them will cause *vasoconstriction*. Stimulating alpha-1 receptors thus will *increase* blood pressure,

Figure 3-1

LOCATION AND EFFECTS OF STIMULATION OF ADRENERGIC RECEPTORS

ALPHA-1 RECEPTORS

Arterioles and Veins: constriction
(epinephrine and norepinephrine)

Glands:
↓ secretions

Eye:
constriction of radial muscle

Intestine:
↓ motility

BETA-1 RECEPTORS

Heart:

↑ heart rate (SA node)

↑ contractility

↑ conduction velocity

↑ automaticity

Kidney:

↑ renin secretion

ALPHA-2 RECEPTORS

CNS Postsynaptic Terminals:

↓ sympathetic outflow from brain

↓ CNS Presynaptic Terminals:
norepinephrine release

↓ Beta Islet Cells of Pancreas: secretion

BETA-2 RECEPTORS

Trachea and Bronchioles: dilation

Pregnant/nonpregnant

Uterus:

relaxation

Arterioles (no beta-2 receptors in skin
or brain):
dilation (epinephrine)

---

while alpha-1 blockers tend to *decrease* blood pressure. Parasympathetic nerves do not significantly innervate peripheral blood vessels.

Alpha-2 receptors are found in the central nervous system. Stimulating them increases their normal function of inhibiting sympathetic outflow from the brain. Thus, alpha-2 agonists reduce blood pressure.

Beta blockers, both *non-cardioselective* (β-1 and β-2), e.g., *propranolol* (Inderal), *timolol* (Blocadren), *nadolol* (Corgard), and β-1 *cardioselective*, e.g., *atenolol* (Tenormin), *metoprolol* (Lopressor, Toprol-XL), *acebutolol* (Sectral), *bisoprolol* (Zebeta), IV *esmolol* (Brevibloc) block the beta-division of the adrenergic (sympathetic) nervous system, reducing heart rate, blood pressure, and the strength of cardiac contraction. These drugs have thus assumed an important role in the management of patients with:

- CAD (by decreasing myocardial oxygen demand), including stable angina pectoris, unstable angina, acute MI (reduce infarct size) and post-MI (reduce recurrent MI and death)

- Hypertension (through decreased cardiac output and decreased renin secretion)

- CHF (blunts cardiotoxic effects of excess circulating catecholamines and improves left ventricular (LV) size and shape [reverse-remodeling])
- Supraventricular and ventricular tachyarrhythmias (increasing refractory period and conduction time of AV node, decreasing automaticity of Purkinje fibers, inhibition of cardiac sympathetic activity)
- Hypertrophic obstructive cardiomyopathy (HOCM) (reducing ventricular contraction force and allowing time for diastolic filling of contracted ventricle thereby reducing LV outflow tract obstruction)
- Mitral valve prolapse (MVP) (inhibits cardiac sympathetic activity)
- Marfan's syndrome and aortic dissection (reduces shear force, blood pressure, and ventricular contractility, and thus slows the rate of aortic dilatation and reduces the risk of rupture)
- Neurocardiogenic syncope (blocks sympathetic increase and intense LV contraction that may precipitate paradoxical vagal reflex)
- Prolonged QT syndrome (beta blockers do not prolong QT interval as do many other drugs)

Drugs that nonselectively antagonize both β-1 and β-2 receptors run the risk of inducing bronchospasm and vasospasm, because β-2 stimulation is important in maintaining bronchodilation and vasodilation. Agents that are "cardioselective" have a greater effect on β-1 (cardiac) adrenoreceptors than on β-2 adrenergic receptors of the bronchi and blood vessels. You should avoid using nonselective beta blockers and use agents with β-1 selectivity cautiously (if at all) in patients with asthma and chronic obstructive pulmonary disease (COPD), since β-1 selectivity is dose dependent, and these drugs become less selective as the dosage is increased. As primary preventive therapy, beta blockers are less effective than other antihypertensive agents at reducing the risk of stroke in older patients with isolated hypertension. In the post-MI setting, beta blockers limit infarct size; suppress ventricular arrhythmias; reduce the incidence of angina, reinfarction, and sudden cardiac death; and improve survival. These agents are effective in slowing the ventricular response in patients with atrial fibrillation or flutter, converting paroxysmal SVT to normal sinus rhythm, and preventing atrial tachyarrhythmias following cardiac surgery.

Beta blockers (e.g. *long-acting metoprolol succinate, carvedilol, bisoprolol*) have been shown to be helpful in prolonging life in carefully treated patients with CHF as well (as do ACE inhibitors/ARBs and the aldosterone antagonists, spironolactone and eplerenone). *Labetalol* (Trandate, Normodyne), either orally or IV, also has α- adrenoreceptor blocking (vasodilating) properties, which makes it particularly useful in patients with hypertensive emergencies or aortic dissection. *Carvedilol* (Coreg), another combined α and nonselective β blocker, is effective in the patient with compensated CHF due to systolic dysfunction. *Nebivolol* (Bystolic), a highly selective β-1 receptor blocker with nitric oxide mediated vasodilating properties, has recently been approved for use in hypertension. Since beta blockers can transiently worsen CHF, these agents should be started at the lowest dose and titrated upward gradually. IV *esmolol* (Brevibloc) is useful in the treatment of SVT and hypertensive emergencies. It has an ultra-short half life of 9 minutes, and therefore is particularly useful in the patient at risk for the common complications of beta blockade.

Potential side effects of beta blockers include:

- Symptomatic bradycardia and heart block
- Exacerbation of Prinzmetal's (vasospastic) angina and cocaine-induced chest pain and/or MI (by inhibiting the vasodilatory β-2 receptor and causing unopposed α-mediated vasoconstriction)
- Peripheral vascular disease (claudication)
- Bronchospasm (asthma)
- Raynaud's phenomenon (by inhibiting β-2 receptors and causing vasoconstriction)
- Lethargy, fatigue, and weight gain
- Decreased libido, impotence
- Disordered sleep patterns, vivid dreams
- Cold hands and feet
- Acute mental disorders, and worsened depression
- Beta blockers may raise triglyceride levels and lower HDL ("good") cholesterol levels.

Highly *lipid soluble* compounds (e.g., *propranolol*) have a high brain penetration, whereas *hydrophilic* compounds (e.g., *atenolol, nadolol*) have a low brain penetration, and theoretically may influence the presence or absence of some of the central nervous system side effects. Furthermore, beta blockers with intrinsic sympathomimetic activity (e.g., *pindolol* [Visken]) have partial agonist activity, and therefore, cause less reduction in cardiac output and heart rate, and negligible peripheral vasoconstriction. Keep in mind that beta blocker therapy should be discontinued by tapering slowly, since sudden withdrawal may lead to a distinct worsening of angina or even an MI (due to excessive catecholamine response). Beta blockers may also potentially mask or exacerbate diabetic hypoglycemia (by increasing beta islet cell insulin secretion), and blunt the catecholamine surge associated with hypoglycemia.

Chapter 4.   Calcium Channel Blockers

Calcium channel blockers block the inward movement of calcium ions across cell membranes, thereby decreasing contractility of vascular smooth muscle cells and cardiac muscle cells, resulting in vasodilatation and decreased cardiac cell contractility (negative inotropic effect). These agents are useful in treating patients with hypertension as well as classic effort and vasospastic angina, by reducing myocardial oxygen demand and increasing myocardial oxygen supply. They include the *dihydropyridines* (*nifedipine* [Procardia, Adalat], *amlodipine* [Norvasc], *felodipine* [Plendil], *isradipine* [DynaCirc], *nicardipine* [Cardene], *nisoldipine* [Sular]), and *clevidipine* [Cleviprex]), which are the more potent vasodilators, and the *nondihydropyridines* (*verapamil* [Isoptin, Calan, Verelan], and *diltiazem* [Cardizem, Tiazac, Dilacor]), which are the less potent vasodilators. Verapamil and diltiazem, in particular, are also useful in treating supraventricular arrhythmias since they also decrease conduction velocity and increase the refractory period of the AV node (by blocking slow inward calcium current).

Controversies regarding the safety of calcium channel blockers emerged during the early 1990s. Administration of the short acting rapid release agents (particularly nifedipine) has been curtailed due to increased cardiovascular mortality witnessed in certain categories of patients. Extended release formulations of the calcium channel blockers (including nifedipine), when indicated, are generally considered effective and safe. Their ability to block calcium-mediated electromechanical coupling in contractile tissue enables these agents to increase blood flow to the heart by dilating the coronary arteries and decreasing oxygen demand by lowering BP, heart rate (e.g., verapamil, diltiazem), and contractility.

Certain calcium channel blockers can be used if anginal symptoms or hypertension are not controlled with beta blockers and ACE inhibitors, or if patients cannot tolerate beta blockers. They do not, however, appear to be universally effective in patients with previous MI, and are not equivalent to beta blockers in post-MI patients. Exception: *Diltiazem* has been demonstrated to be helpful in preventing recurrent MI, but only after non ST segment elevation MI in those with good LV function. Furthermore, short-acting first generation calcium channel blockers (e.g., *nifedipine*) have been implicated in increased morbidity and mortality (in the setting of acute MI) and should not be used. Rate-slowing agents (e.g., diltiazem, verapamil) can be useful in patients with supraventricular tachyarrhythmias (e.g., SVT, atrial fibrillation or flutter).

Aggressive BP reduction can cause myocardial and cerebral ischemia and/ or infarction. Short-acting preparations (particularly SL or oral nifedipine) may worsen ischemia (by lowering blood pressure and reflexly increasing heart rate), cause excessive hypotension and stroke, and should be avoided. Long-acting agents should be used. An exception is intravenous clevidipine, an ultra short acting dihydropyridine with little to no reflex tachycardia, approved for use in severe hypertension. In general, calcium channel blockers should not be used alone to treat stable angina pectoris unless there is a clear contraindication for beta blockers or nitrates. However, patients with variant (Prinzmetal's) angina (where vasoconstriction is the predominant mechanism of myocardial ischemia) are best treated with nitrates and calcium channel blockers, since *beta blockers may worsen coronary spasm (due to unopposed alpha vasoconstriction) in Prinzmetal's angina.* Calcium channel blockers are useful as first line agents in these patients.

Since verapamil and diltiazem can induce significant bradycardia, they should be used with caution if a beta blocker is part of the regimen.

Verapamil (by depressing myocardial contractility) can be helpful in selected patients with hypertrophic obstructive cardiomyopathy (HOCM).

Calcium channel blockers may be preferred in patients with COPD, pulmonary hypertension, peripheral vascular disease, Raynaud's phenomenon, or SVT.

The afterload-reducing effect of extended release nifedipine may delay the need for aortic valve replacement in patients with aortic regurgitation (AR). Frequent or adverse side effects of calcium channel blockers include dizziness, headache, gingival hyperplasia, bradycardia and AV block (verapamil, diltiazem), flushing, constipation (verapamil) and precipitation of CHF in patients with marginal LV function. In otherwise well-treated patients with CHF, *amlodipine* is more "vascular selective" and may be cautiously added if essential (e.g., for control of hypertension). Currently amlodipine and felodipine have the safest "track-record" in patients with LV systolic dysfunction.

Verapamil can raise digoxin levels and precipitate digitalis toxicity.

Keep in mind that peripheral edema can occur as a side effect of calcium channel blockers (and therefore should not be confused with a sign of CHF).

In patients with diabetic hypertension, ACE inhibitors and ARBs, along with calcium channel blocker therapy (particularly dihydropyridines) have been shown to be effective.

Chapter 5. Nitrates

Sublingual, oral, cutaneous, and parenteral nitrates have been the mainstay of treatment for patients with stable and unstable angina pectoris due to atherosclerotic CAD, coronary artery spasm (Prinzmetal's angina), and acute MI. By conversion to nitric oxide (NO), also known as endothelium derived relaxing factor, organic nitrates stimulate formation of cyclic guanosine monophosphate (GMP) which mediates vascular smooth muscle cell relaxation. (**Figure 5-1**)

Figure 5-1. Mechanism of action of organic nitrates.

These agents induce coronary vasodilation (including dilation at sites of coronary artery stenoses) and dilate peripheral veins, thereby reducing venous return to the heart, and thus decrease heart size, which lowers myocardial oxygen demand. Nitrates lessen symptoms of CHF and, in combination with hydralazine (a peripheral vasodilator), improve survival and delay progression of LV dysfunction (although not as well as ACE inhibitors). Despite their extensive

Figure 5-1

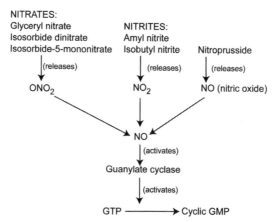

ORGANIC NITRATES - MECHANISM OF ACTION

NITRATES:
Glyceryl nitrate
Isosorbide dinitrate
Isosorbide-5-mononitrate

NITRITES:
Amyl nitrite
Isobutyl nitrite

Nitroprusside

(releases) → ONO_2

(releases) → NO_2

(releases) → NO (nitric oxide)

NO

(activates)

Guanylate cyclase

(activates)

GTP ⟶ Cyclic GMP

Cyclic GMP vasodilates arteries and veins by decreasing intracellular Ca^{++}, resulting in muscle cell relaxation.(GTP = guanosine triphosphate; GMP = guanosine monophosphate)

17

"track-record" in relieving symptoms and improving exercise tolerance and the quality of life for patients with coronary artery disease (CAD), there is no evidence that nitrates reduce mortality. Nitroglycerin is available as a *SL tablet* (e.g., Nitrostat) or *spray* (Nitrolingual) to shorten or prevent an anticipated angina attack, *long-acting oral tablets* (e.g., *isosorbide dinitrate* [Isordil], *mononitrate* [Ismo, Imdur, Monoket], *topical ointment* (e.g., Nitro-Bid 2%) or *patch* (e.g., Nitro-Dur, Transderm-Nitro, Minitran), as well as an *IV preparation* (e.g., Tridil). If angina occurs under predictable circumstances (e.g., taking a walk, climbing a flight of stairs), nitroglycerin can be used prophylactically before the activity to prevent it from occurring. Nitrates decrease the heart's demand for oxygen by reducing preload and increase blood supply by relaxing the coronary arteries.

Keep in mind that all nitrates are subject to "tolerance", i.e., with continuous use their effects may wane or even disappear. Eccentric dosage schedules with a "nitrate-free interval" of 8–10 hours is generally recommended to preserve efficacy in long-term treatment. Transdermal nitroglycerin preparations, although initially greeted with enthusiasm, are being replaced, for the most part, by extended-release oral preparations. Use nitroglycerin with caution in patients with acute inferior MI with RV involvement. (Patients with RV infarction have a stiff, noncompliant ventricle that depends on high filling pressures; thus, these patients may not tolerate the reduction in preload or venodilation induced by these medications.) Do not administer nitroglycerin to patients who present with an ACS, including unstable angina, who have used phosphodiesterase-5 (PDE-5) inhibitors for erectile dysfunction e.g., *sildenafil* (Viagra), *vardenafil* (Levitra), or *tadalafil* (Cialis) within the previous 24-48 hours. These agents are also vasodilators and marked and potentially dangerous hypotension may result with resultant myocardial ischemia. Other problems with nitroglycerin include the fact that 10% of patients do not respond and another 10% have associated intolerable headaches that may necessitate discontinuation. Patients who have frequent angina, or angina at night (during the nitrate-free period) should be treated with a second drug (e.g., beta blocker, calcium channel blocker).

Chapter 6.   Angiotensin Converting Enzyme (ACE) Inhibitors

The renin-angiotensin-aldosterone system plays an important role in regulating blood pressure and maintaining cardiovascular homeostasis (balance). Drugs that act on this system (e.g., ACE inhibitors, ARBs) are of great value in cardiology (**Figure 6-1**).

The enzyme renin is secreted into the bloodstream by the juxtaglomerular cells of the kidney in response to decreased renal blood flow and increased sympathetic nervous system (beta-1 adrenergic) activity (as may occur in CHF). Renin then acts to convert angiotensinogen (from the liver) to the inactive precursor, angiotensin I. Angiotensin converting enzyme (ACE) in the pulmonary capillaries facilitates the conversion of angiotensin I to active angiotensin II, a potent vasoconstrictor and stimulator of aldosterone secretion by the adrenal cortex (aldosterone promotes absorption of sodium from the distal nephron), which raises arterial blood pressure and improves cardiac output and renal blood flow, thus turning off the renin-activated system.

These "compensatory" mechanisms, however, can have deleterious effects in the failing heart. Excessive vasoconstriction increases peripheral vascular resistance (increases afterload) which can decrease LV function and cardiac output, and salt and water retention by the kidney can worsen the already elevated ventricular filling pressure (increases preload).

Figure 6-1. The renin-angiotensin-aldosterone system and sites of drug intervention. Blockade of the renin-angiotensin-aldosterone system can take place at five pivotal sites: (1) Inhibiting the release of renin from the juxtaglomerular cells of the kidney with beta-adrenergic blockers; (2) Blocking the activity of renin with direct renin inhibitors; (3) Blocking the conversion of angiotensin I to angiotensin II with ACE inhibitors; (4) Blocking the AT type I receptor with ARBs; and (5) Antagonizing the effects of aldosterone at the distal renal tubule with aldosterone antagonists. **Note:** Unlike ACE inhibitors, the ARBs do not affect serum bradykinin levels and, therefore, cough is not a common side effect.

ACE inhibitors, by preventing the conversion of angiotensin I to angiotensin II, reduce systemic blood pressure by promoting vasodilation, and reduce sodium reabsorption from the distal nephron. These agents also increase levels of bradykinin and vasodilatory prostaglandins. By reducing peripheral vascular resistance (decreasing afterload) ACE inhibitors reduce the stress (impedance) to the heart and increase cardiac output in heart failure. They are also useful as antihypertensive agents.

Figure 6-1

RENIN-ANGIOTENSIN-ALDOSTERONE SYSTEM AND SITES OF DRUG INTERVENTION

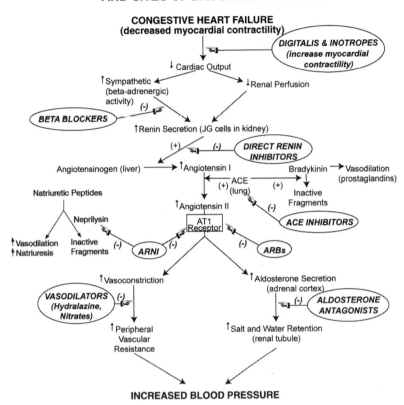

ACE inhibitors include *captopril* (Capoten), *enalapril* (Vasotec), *lisinopril* (Zestril, Prinivil), *ramipril* (Altace), *fosinopril* (Monopril), *quinapril* (Accupril), *benazepril* (Lotensin), and *trandolapril* (Mavik). These vasodilators are the mainstay of therapy for patients with CHF due to LV systolic dysfunction (reduces mortality and hospitalization in patients with symptomatic CHF and in those who are asymptomatic with poor LV function). While treating hypertension, they help provide renoprotection in patients with diabetes and proteinuria.

They are useful in decreasing morbidity and mortality in patients with acute MI (with EF < 40%). Therapy should be started early in stable, high-risk patients, e.g., anterior MI, previous MI, Killip class II (S3 gallop, rales, radiographic CHF). After load reduction with an ACE inhibitor is of value in the management of chronic AR. Side effects may include

- Hypotension
- Worsening of renal function with volume or salt depletion or concomitant use of diuretics
- Hyperkalemia in patients with renal dysfunction (particularly diabetics) and in those receiving potassium supplements or potassium-sparing diuretics
- Acute renal failure in patients with bilateral renal artery stenosis (or stenosis in the artery to a solitary kidney).
- Cough, loss of taste, rash, or rarely angioneurotic edema.

To minimize the hypotension risk in diuretic treated patients, diuretics should either be held or reduced in dose (if possible) before starting ACE inhibitor therapy. You should exercise caution in volume depleted or hyponatremic patients. Keep in mind that a bothersome dry *cough* (which may relate to increased bradykinin levels) may result, which at times can be mistaken for the symptoms of CHF. Since ACE inhibitors can impair renal function, the BUN, creatinine and serum potassium levels should be monitored. Hyperkalemia may occur especially if ACE inhibitors a reused with other drugs that increase potassium (e.g., potassium sparing diuretics), and if renal insufficiency is present. Mild increases in potassium may be tolerated; however, significant increases are indications to discontinue the drug. These agents should not be used by pregnant women.

Chapter 7.   Angiotensin Receptor Blockers (ARBs)

Angiotensin receptor blockers (ARBs), e.g., *losartan* (Cozaar), *candesartan* (Atacand), *irbesartan* (Avapro), and *valsartan* (Diovan), *olmesartan* (Benicar), *telmisartan* (Micardis), *eprosartan* (Teveten), and *azilsartan* (Edarbi) specifically block the angiotensin II receptor AT1 which causes effective blockade of the renin-angiotensin system. These agents act at a different site from ACE inhibitors to block the effects of angiotensin II and theoretically have the benefits of ACE inhibition, except formation of bradykinin, and without adverse side effects, particularly cough (**Figure 6-1**). ARBs represent a major breakthrough in the management of hypertension and CHF and are now being used more often (at least in ACE-intolerant patients). **Note:** although ARBs are clearly better tolerated than ACE inhibitors, producing a far smaller incidence of cough or angioneurotic edema, it should not be expected that renal insufficiency, hypotension, or hyperkalemia will occur less frequently with ARBs compared with ACE inhibitors. As with ACE inhibitors, to minimize the hypotensive risk in diuretic treated patients, diuretics should be held or reduced (if possible) before using ARBs. These agents should not be taken by pregnant women. Caution is advised when considering these agents if a history of ACE inhibitor angioedema is present.

Chapter 8.   Angiotensin Receptor Neprilysin Inhibitors

A new class of drug called angiotensin receptor neprilysin inhibitor (ARNI), which combines an ARB (valsartan) with a neprilysin inhibitor (sacubitril), marketed as Entresto, has been shown to be superior to an ACE inhibitor (enalapril) in reducing cardiovascular mortality and hospitalization in patients with CHF. The drugs ability to block the renin-angiotensin system and inhibit the enzymatic breakdown of endogenous natriuretic and vasodilatory peptides provides a novel approach to the treatment of CHF. Of note, symptomatic hypotension is more common with an ARNI than with an ACE inhibitor or ARB. Caution should be used when initiating an ARNI in patients with hypotension or kidney impairment. If switching from an ACE inhibitor, allow a 36 hour washout period between administration of drugs. Administration of an ARNI is contraindicated with pregnancy, concomitant use of an ACE inhibitor, concomitant aliskerin use in patients with diabetes mellitus, or previous angioedema with an ACE inhibitor or ARB. (**Figure 6-1**)

Chapter 9. Direct Renin Inhibitors

Aliskiren (Tekturna) is the first direct renin inhibitor approved by the FDA for treatment of hypertension, either alone or in combination with other antihypertensive agents. Unlike ACE inhibitors and ARBs, which target the renin-angiotensin-aldosterone system at later stages, direct renin inhibitors, e.g., aliskiren, target the renin-angiotensin-aldosterone system at the first and rate-limiting step. By blocking the action of renin, this agent decreases the production of angiotensin and aldosterone, and thus reduces systemic blood pressure by promoting vasodilation and reducing sodium retention from the distal renal tubule. (**Figure 6-1**) Direct inhibition of renin does not increase bradykinin levels thought to be responsible for the angioedema and cough seen with ACE inhibitors. These agents should not be used by pregnant women. Results of long-term clinical outcome studies are needed to establish the precise role of this novel class of antihypertensive medication.

Chapter 10. Inotropic Agents

Digitalis Glycosides

The digitalis glycosides inhibit the Na^+-K^+ ATPase pump in myocardial cell membranes. This increases intracellular sodium (and extracellular potassium) which, in turn, increases intracellular calcium (by sodium-calcium exchanger) which increases the force of myocardial contraction.

Figure 10-1. Digitalis—Mechanism of action.

By its unique combination of increasing the force of ventricular contractions (positive inotropic effect) and decreasing the ventricular rate in SVTs (vagally-induced inhibition of AV nodal conduction and sympatholytic effects), *digoxin* (Lanoxin) is particularly useful in the treatment of patients with CHF due to impaired LV systolic function, especially when atrial fibrillation, flutter, and other

Figure 10-1

DIGITALIS - MECHANISM OF ACTION

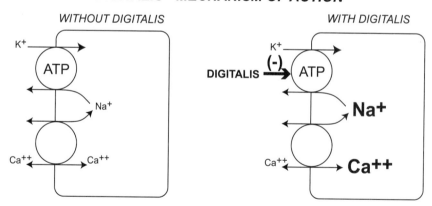

Digitalis inhibits the myocardial cell ATPase pump. Intracellular $[Na^+]$ rises. This causes intracellular $[Ca^{++}]$ to rise. Ca^{++} increases muscle cell contractility.

Note: Acute digitalis toxicity can cause *hyper*kalemia (digoxin blocks the Na^+ K^+ ATPase pump, so more K^+ remains outside the cells), but *hypo*kalemia can predispose to chronic digitals toxicity (digoxin competes with K^+ for the same ATPase binding site, so more digoxin is available to exert its effects).

atrial tachyarrhythmias are also present. In patients with stable mild to moderate heart failure and substantial LV systolic dysfunction (ejection fraction $\leq 35\%$) the withdrawal of digoxin from triple therapy (i.e., ACE inhibitor, diuretic, digitalis) results in clinical deterioration. Although long-term prospective data show that digoxin decreases hospitalization, it does not confer added mortality benefit as do beta blockers, ACE inhibitors and spironolactone; therefore its use in normal sinus rhythm remains optional. For patients with significant symptomatic LV systolic dysfunction, digoxin provides benefit when digoxin levels are 0.5 to 1.0 ng/ml. The therapeutic-toxic window is narrow. Data suggests that patients with serum digoxin levels of 1.0–2.0 ng/ml (previously regarded at "therapeutic") and women (who tend to have higher serum levels on fixed doses of digoxin than men) have an increased mortality risk. Serum digoxin levels are particularly valuable in assessing patients suspected of having digitalis toxicity. However, the serum digoxin level is not a substitute for a complete clinical assessment of the patient. Patients with hypoxemia, hypokalemia, and hypomagnesemia, for example, may have toxic manifestations of digitalis excess even in the absence of an elevated serum digoxin concentration.

Digitalis toxicity: Despite the best of intentions, patients often make inadvertent medication errors (especially the elderly). For example, a patient may take a certain medication, e.g., digoxin, several times a day, thinking that it was a different medication and wonders why he or she is becoming nauseated! Common early clues to digitalis intoxication include GI complaints (e.g., nausea, vomiting, anorexia), along with visual disturbances (e.g., blurred, yellow-green and/or halo vision), electrolyte abnormalities (e.g., hyperkalemia), and neurologic symptoms and/or signs (e.g., headache; fatigue, disorientation, delirium, and confusion). Cardiac arrhythmias are additional clues to digitalis toxicity. These include PVCs, paroxysmal atrial tachycardia with AV block, bidirectional VT (QRS complexes from two different ectopic foci alternate in morphology), "regularization" of atrial fibrillation (regular R-R intervals). Gynecomastia is a rare sequela. Digitalis toxicity is frequently seen in advancing age, renal insufficiency, diuretic use, hypothyroidism or accidental/deliberate overdose. Therapy for digoxin toxicity generally requires simply withholding the drug and monitoring the patient. Tachyarrhythmias can be treated with antiarrhythmic agents e.g., lidocaine (Xylocaine), phenytoin (Dilantin), and beta blockers. Hypokalemia can precipitate this condition and therefore should be corrected. Keep in mind that amiodarone, verapamil, and quinidine can raise digoxin levels and increase the risk of digitalis toxicity. Life-threatening digitalis intoxication requires immediate attention and can be treated with digoxin-specific antibodies, e.g., Digibind.

Sympathomimetic Amines (e.g., Dopamine, Dobutamine)

When additional inotropic support is needed in the treatment of CHF, intravenous sympathomimetic amines (e.g., *dopamine* [Intropin], *dobutamine* [Dobutrex]) and phosphodiesterase inhibitors (e.g., milrinone [Primacor]) may be administered, usually as a short-term continuous infusion. Their hemo-dynamic effect is to shift a depressed ventricular performance (Frank-Starling) curve in an upward direction, so that for a given ventricular filling pressure, stroke volume and cardiac output are increased (**Figure 10-2**).

Figure 10-2. Ventricular function (Frank-Starling) curves in a normal person and a patient with CHF relating cardiac output (a measure of LV performance) to left ventricular end-diastolic pressure (LVEDP) or volume (preload). In heart failure, the curve is displaced downward, so that at a given LVEDP, the cardiac output is lower than in a normal individual. Diuretics and venodilators (e.g., nitrates) reduce LVEDP (preload), but do not change the position of the curve; the output is still low. Pulmonary congestion improves, but cardiac output may fall. Inotropic therapy and afterload reduction (e.g., vasodilator therapy) displaces the curve upward toward normal so that at any LVEDP, the cardiac output is higher. Radiographically evident pulmonary redistribution and edema correlate with elevated LVEDP as noted.

Intravenous dopamine and dobutamine are commonly used sympathomimetic amines in the treatment of acute CHF. At low doses (2–5 ug/kg/min), dopamine has primarily a renal vasodilating action (dopaminergic effect), and may selectively improve renal blood flow and promote diuresis in oliguric patients. At moderate doses (5–10 ug/kg/min), the inotropic (β-1 agonist) effect of dopamine predominates, and at high doses, its primary action is vasoconstriction (α agonist effect). Dopamine may increase pulmonary capillary wedge pressure and should be reserved, therefore, for the patient with significant hypotension. If the patient is normotensive or only mildly hypotensive, dobutamine is the preferred inotropic agent.

Figure 10-2

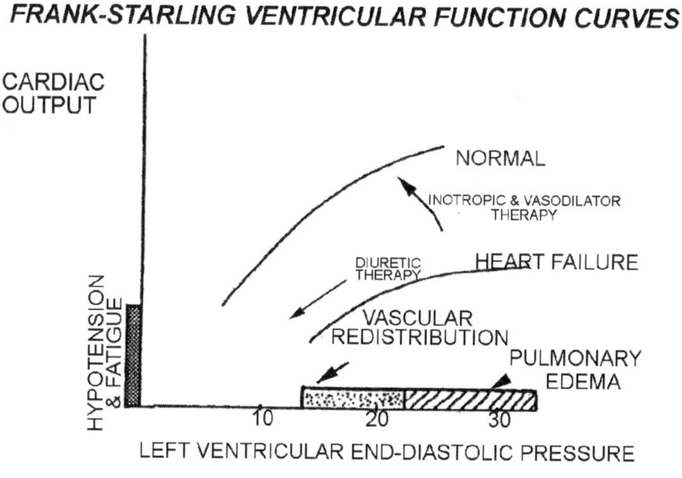

FRANK-STARLING VENTRICULAR FUNCTION CURVES

Dobutamine primarily stimulates cardiac β-1 receptors with little α or β-2 adrenergic activity and has the advantage of having less chronotropic effect than dopamine. Doses of 2.5–15 ug/kg/min lead to an increase in cardiac output without a marked increase in peripheral vascular resistance or heart rate. Dobutamine should not be used alone, however, if the patient is markedly hypotensive since it has minimal vasoconstrictive activity. As a result, it causes a fall in systemic arterial and pulmonary capillary wedge pressure. The combination of low dose dopamine with dobutamine improves myocardial contractility, maintains systemic blood pressure, enhances renal blood flow and reduces pulmonary capillary wedge pressure and thus may be an extremely effective regimen.

Phosphodiesterase Inhibitors (e.g., Amrinone, Milrinone)

Tachyphylaxis (rapidly decreasing response after a few doses) to the hemodynamic effects of dobutamine can occur after 2 to 3 days of continuous therapy and may require either increasing the drug dose or switching to another intravenous inotrope, i.e., a phosphodiesterase-3 inhibitor e.g., *milrinone* (Primacor), *amrinone* (Inocor). Inhibiting phosphodiesterase in cardiac muscle and smooth muscle of peripheral vessels with milrinone preserves intracellular cyclic adenosine monophosphate (cAMP) which results in enhanced myocardial contraction (positive inotropic effect) and peripheral vasodilation (vasodilator effect), the so-called "inodilator" effect. Cardiac output and stroke volume increase while pulmonary capillary wedge pressure and peripheral vascular resistance decrease due to mixed cardiac and vascular effects. Milrinone appears to be more potent than amrinone and has less major adverse side effects (e.g., thrombocytopenia). Since these drugs cause vasodilation, hypotension may be aggravated and can be a limiting factor. As with sympathomimetics, these drugs can cause mild tachycardia and aggravation of ventricular arrhythmias.

There can be surprisingly different hemodynamic responses to dobutamine and milrinone in individual patients, with much greater increase of cardiac output when switching from one to the other. Although intermittent intravenous inotropic therapy in advanced CHF patients has been shown to increase physical capacity, there is concern for aggravated arrhythmias and sudden death. Since quality of life is often the issue more than quantity of life in these patients, intermittent inotropic treatment may be a reasonable option.

Chapter 11.   Diuretics

Diuretics are a mainstay in the treatment of hypertension and CHF. In CHF, they help to eliminate excess sodium and water through renal excretion and can ease shortness of breath (due to pulmonary congestion) and swelling (due to peripheral edema) within hours or days, whereas other agents (e.g., digitalis, vasodilators) may take weeks or even months. In hypertension, diuretics act, in part, by elimination of intravascular volume. Because the compensatory response to most other classes of antihypertensive medications involves sodium retention, diuretics can lead to improved blood pressure control. The three most commonly used groups of diuretics are the thiazide diuretics, loop diuretics, and potassium-sparing diuretics. A new class of diuretics currently under evaluation are the aquaretics ("vaptans"). (**Figure 11-1**) These classes can be distinguished by their site of action in the kidney tubule, their mechanism, and form of diuresis that they elicit (solute vs. water diuresis [i.e., aquaresis]).

Figure 11-1. Sites of action of diuretics. Thiazide diuretics inhibit sodium and chloride reabsorption in the distal convoluted tubule. Loop diuretics inhibit

Figure 11-1

DIURETICS AND THEIR SITES OF ACTION

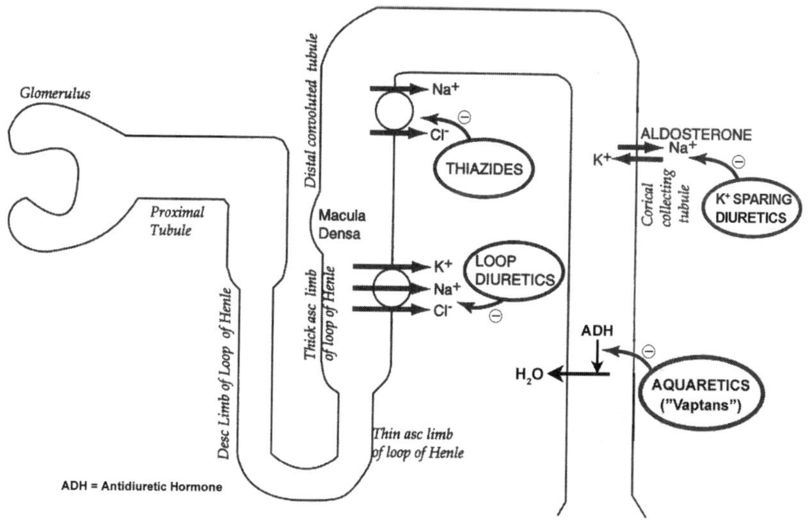

sodium, potassium, and chloride reabsorption in the thick ascending limb of the loop of Henle. Potassium sparing diuretics inhibit potassium secretion and influence sodium excretion in the cortical collecting tubule. Aquaretics, also known as vasopressin antagonists ("vaptans"), are now being used in the treatment of euvolemic or hypervolemic hyponatremia. These agents block the antidiuretic (water retaining) effects of vasopressin on the renal collecting duct, resulting in an increase in solute-free water excretion, along with an increase in serum sodium concentration.

Thiazides

Thiazides, e.g., *hydrochlorothiazide* (HydroDIURIL), *chlorothiazide* (Diuril), *chlorthalidone* (Hygroton), and *indapamide* (Lozol), act on the distal renal tubule and collecting segment and are standard therapy for chronic CHF when edema is mild to modest, either alone or in combination with loop diuretics. These agents are less potent than loop diuretics, but because of their longer duration of action, are beneficial in chronic conditions, e.g., mild to moderate CHF (except in patients with renal dysfunction, i.e., serum creatinine level > 2 mg/dL). Thiazides are also useful in treating hypertension. Chlorthalidone is stronger and longer acting than hydrochlorothiazide, and due to its superior clinical outcome data, may be the preferred agent in controlling hypertension.

Loop Diuretics

With more advanced degrees of CHF the stronger loop diuretics, which impair absorption in the thick ascending limb of the loop of Henle, and/or combinations of diuretics, e.g., thiazide or a thiazide-like agent *metolazone* (Zaroxolyn, Diulo) and a loop diuretic e.g., *furosemide* (Lasix), *bumetanide* (Bumex), *torsemide* (Demadex) may be needed. Both these agents administered together tend to be effective even in the setting of impaired renal function. A more prominent natriuretic effect results than with either agent alone since they act on different segments of the renal tubule ("sequential nephron block"). Thiazide diuretics alone are ineffective in the setting of diminished renal function (when the serum creatinine is >2.5 mg/dL). Loop diuretics e.g., furosemide (Lasix), bumetanide (Bumex), torsemide (Demadex), all sulfonamide derivatives, are effective in patients with renal insufficiency and CHF and/or hypertension. *Ethacrynic acid* (Edecrin), a non-sulfonamide derivative, is useful in patients allergic to sulfa drugs (but is more ototoxic). Intravenous loop diuretics are of great value in the acute management of pulmonary edema. In addition to its diuretic effect, and even preceding it, these drugs may induce venodilation (by promoting prostaglandin and nitric oxide release from endothelial cells which act to relax vascular smooth muscle), and thereby decrease venous return and reduce pulmonary congestion.

Potassium Sparing Diuretics

Potassium sparing diuretics, e.g., *spironolactone* (Aldactone), *triamterene* (Dyrenium), and *amiloride* (Midamor), are relatively weak diuretics that are useful when maintenance of serum potassium is crucial. These drugs are rarely used alone and are often combined with thiazide or loop diuretics to offset urinary potassium loss. Spironolactone (Aldactone) is an aldosterone antagonist that acts on the aldosterone-sensitive region of the cortical collecting tubule. When added to an ACE inhibitor and a loop diuretic, with or without digoxin, this agent has been shown to improve CHF symptoms and reduce mortality rates by competitively inhibiting the adverse effects of aldosterone on *myocardial remodeling* (i.e., the process whereby the failing heart undergoes changes in LV size, shape, and thickness to maintain adequate forward flow). The other potassium-sparing agents e.g., dyrenium and amiloride act independently of aldosterone.

Diuretic effects should be monitored carefully since excessive administration may result in a drop in cardiac output, hypotension and prerenal azotemia. The most common side effects of the thiazide and loop diuretics include intravascular volume depletion, hypokalemia and hypomagnesemia (which predisposes to ventricular arrhythmias), metabolic alkalosis, weakness, fatigue, sexual dysfunction, elevated lipid levels (increased LDL cholesterol and triglyceride levels), hyperuricemia (and possible precipitation of gout) due to decreased clearance of uric acid, and hyperglycemia (because of impaired pancreatic insulin release and/ or decreased peripheral glucose utilization). The most serious potential adverse effects of the potassium sparing diuretics is the development of hyperkalemia, resulting from impaired excretion of potassium. Spironolactone also possesses antiandrogenic activity and may produce gynecomastia in men. Newer aldosterone antagonists, e.g., *eplerenone* (Inspra), have been shown to improve survival in post-MI patients with LV systolic dysfunction and CHF. These agents may reduce some of the side effects associated with aldosterone (e.g., gynecomastia) while providing a diuretic and potassium conserving activity similar to that of spironolactone.

Chapter 12. Antiplatelet Agents

Aspirin

Aspirin (acetylsalicylic acid) is the most widely used antiplatelet agent in cardiology. This simple, over-the-counter pill, has proved to be a cornerstone of therapy for patients with atherosclerotic vascular disease. If an individual has already had a heart attack or stroke, a daily dose of aspirin will substantially reduce the odds of another event or even death from cardiovascular disease. Furthermore, aspirin dramatically improves survival for patients in the throes of an MI. *The use of just one aspirin tablet chewed (or swallowed) at the onset of symptoms of a heart attack can cause a 25% reduction in the incidence of MI or death. Keep in mind that nitroglycerin, although it may relieve anginal pain, does not prevent a heart attack or save lives.* Moreover, in patients with stable angina pectoris without a history of acute MI, aspirin lessens the occurrence of subsequent MI and mortality. As with all medications, however, any benefit must be weighed against risk. In the case of aspirin, these risks include bleeding into the brain or GI tract (especially in older patients). Those who have active peptic ulcer disease, consume > 2 alcoholic beverages a day, have severe uncontrolled hypertension, or are taking blood thinners, e.g., warfarin (Coumadin) are at high risk for bleeding.Although aspirin plays an important role in secondary prevention, i.e., in patients with known ischemic vascular disease, it is not recommended that otherwise healthy individuals who are not at high risk, especially those > age 70, should routinely take aspirin for cardiovascular protection. The decision to use aspirin, particularly for primary prevention (i.e., in individuals without a history of CAD), should be made on a case-by-case basis, weighing the patient's risk of bleeding against potential benefit.

Platelets play a key pathophysiologic role in the development of the atherosclerotic plaque and the acute phase of coronary thrombosis. By irreversible inhibition of the cyclooxygenase enzyme, aspirin prevents platelet production of thromboxane A2, a vasoconstrictor and an important substance for induction of platelet aggregation. (**Figure 12-1**)

Figure 12-1.Pathways to thrombosis and sites of drug intervention. After disruption of a vulnerable atherosclerotic plaque, tissue factor and subendothelial collagen are exposed, which initiates platelet activation and aggregation (white clot pathway) and the coagulation cascade (red clot pathway), ultimately resulting in a fibrin clot. Antiplatelet drugs interfere with platelet function at various sites along the platelet activation and aggregation pathway. Aspirin irreversibly inhibits

Figure 12-1

PATHWAYS TO THROMBOSIS
AND SITES OF DRUG INTERVENTION

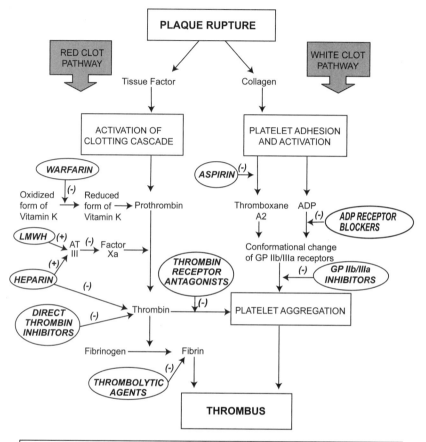

Note: *ADP Receptor Blockers:* clopidogrel, prasugrel, ticagrelor; *Glycoprotein (GP) IIb/IIIa inhibitors:* abciximab, eptifibatide, tirofiban ; *Low molecular weight heparin (LMWH):* enoxaparin, fragmin; *Direct thrombin inhibitors:* bivalirudin, lepirudin, argatroban; *Thrombolytic agents:* tPA, rPA, TNK-tPA; AT III = Antithrombin III; Factor Xa = Activated Factor X; ADP = Adenosine Diphosphate

cyclooxygenase and thus decreases platelet production of thromboxane A2, an important activator of platelets. Thienopyridines (e.g., clopidogrel, ticlopidine, prasugrel) and nonthienopyridines (e.g. ticagrelor) inhibit the binding of adenosine diphosphate (ADP) to the P2Y12 platelet receptor, which also blocks platelet activation. Thrombin receptor antagonists (e.g., vorapaxar) inhibit the binding of thrombin to the protease-activated receptor, PAR-1, on the platelet surface, which blocks platelet aggregation. Glycoprotein (GP) IIb/IIIa inhibitors (abciximab, eptifibatide, tirofiban) block fibrinogen binding to the platelet GP IIb/IIIa receptor and thus block the critical and final common pathway to platelet aggregation. Anticoagulant drugs interfere with the coagulation factors at various sites along the clotting cascade. Unfractionated heparin and low molecular weight hep arin (LMWH), combined with their cofactor antithrombin III (AT III), both inhibit thrombin activation from prothrombin. Unfractionated heparin inhibits factor Xa and thrombin to a similar degree, whereas LMWH inhibits factor Xa more potently than it inhibits thrombin. Factor Xa inhibitors, both indirect (e.g., fondaparinux) which binds with AT III, and direct (e.g., rivaroxaban, apixaban, edoxaban), selectively inactivate factor Xa, and indirectly inhibit thrombin generation. Direct thrombin inhibitors (bivalirudin, lepirudin, argatroban) predominantly inhibit thrombin itself. Warfarin inhibits the formation of reduced vitamin K and thus decreases production of functional pro-thrombin. Thrombolytic agents (e.g., tPA, rPA, TNK-tPA) convert plasminogen to plasmin, thereby activating the endogenous fibrinolytic system. These agents lyse fibrin and dissolve occlusive clots that have already formed.

The clinical benefits for aspirin have been shown in patients with acute and chronic CAD, post-CABG (lowers the likelihood of graft occlusion), PCI (prevents thrombotic complications following coronary stenting), nonvalvular atrial fibrillation, prosthetic valves, and transient ischemic attacks (TIAs) (reduces the risk of stroke). In acute coronary syndrome (ACS), aspirin alone has been shown to be effective in reducing acute MI in patients with unstable angina as well as augmenting the benefit of heparin (by reducing the incidence for post-heparin rebound thrombosis). Similarly, in acute ST elevation MI, aspirin alone reduces the risk for adverse events when combined with thrombolytic therapy. Of note, dipyridamole, a relatively weak platelet inhibitor, in combination with low dose aspirin (marketed as Aggrenox) has been shown to be superior to as-pirin monotherapy, but not more effective than clopidogrel alone, in preventing recurrent stroke.

Despite its widespread use, the optimal dose of aspirin has not been established. According to previous practice guidelines, higher doses (162–325 mg) of aspi-rin are recommended immediately in patients with ACS (preferably non-enteric coated and chewed for rapid absorption), and for at least 1 month, and up to 3–6 months, in patients undergoing PCI with a bare metal or drug eluting stent respec-tively, followed by a lower dose (75–162 mg) of aspirin daily thereafter. More recent studies, however, have shown that lower doses of aspirin are safer and as effective as higher doses for reducing the risk of cardiovascular events. Accord-ingly, updated guidelines recommend a low dose (81 mg) of aspirin indefinitely in most patients with acute or chronic ischemic vascular disease, including those who have undergone PCI, unless specifically contraindicated. In special circum-stances, e.g., post-CABG, a higher maintenance dose (325 mg) of aspirin may be preferable (at least for the first year) to help maintain graft patency.

Adenosine Diphosphate (ADP) Receptor Antagonists (e.g., Clopidogrel, Ticlopidine, Prasugrel, Ticagrelor, Cangrelor)

If aspirin use is contraindicated (because of hypersensitivity or intolerance), *clopi-dogrel* (Plavix), a thienopyridine that irreversibly inhibits the binding of adenosine diphosphate (ADP) to the P2Y12 receptor on platelets, should be considered (**Figure 12-1**). Clopidogrel inhibits ADP-induced platelet aggregation and has been shown to have favorable effects on cardiovascular events (particularly in combination with aspirin, on reducing the incidence of stent thrombosis) and does not present the hematologic complications (e.g., neutropenia, thrombotic thrombocytopenic purpura) associated with *ticlopidine* (Ticlid), an older thienopyridine. The combination of clopidogrel, the most widely used agent in this class, plus aspirin (indefinitely), so-called dual antiplatelet therapy (DAPT), provides benefit in patients with unstable angina, non ST elevation MI, ST elevation MI (when combined with fibrinolytic therapy), and in those with stable CAD or ACS who undergo coronary stent implantation. The optimal loading dose, timing, and duration of clopidogrel therapy, however, remains unresolved. To achieve effective levels of platelet inhibition more rapidly, a standard loading dose of 300 mg of clopidogrel, followed by a daily maintenance dose of 75 mg is recommended. Compared to the conventional loading dose of 300 mg, a loading dose of 600 mg provides even faster and higher degrees of platelet inhibition, without a significant increase in bleeding, and is currently being used in many centers. In addition to aspirin, in patients with stable CAD, updated guidelines recommended a minimum of 1 month of clopidogrel therapy after bare metal stenting (BMS). and at least 6 months after newer generation drug eluting stent (DES) implantation. In patients with ACS, at least 12 months of clopidogrel therapy is recommended, with or without a coronary stent (BMS or DES), to reduce the risk of future MI and stent thrombosis in patients who are not at high risk for bleeding. Although clopidogrel has been shown to be of benefit if started prior to PCI, a minority of patients will require CABG, which makes the "upstream" use of clopidogrel (i.e., before catheterization) somewhat problematic (due to concerns it will delay surgery or increase the risk of bleeding). Clopidogrel should be discontinued at least 5 days prior to CABG to allow for its antiplatelet effect to wear off and to minimize the risk of perioperative bleeding. It may be prudent, therefore, to wait until the coronary anatomy is identified and decisions about revascularization (PCI vs. CABG) are made before initiating clopidogrel treatment. Of note, not all patients respond to clopidogrel with similar benefit. Clopidogrel is a prodrug that requires hepatic metabolism to its active form by the cytochrome P 450 (CYP) enzymatic system, particularly CYP2C19. Patients on clopidogrel who carry a reduced-function allele of the CYP2C19 gene, especially those taking a proton pump inhibitor, e.g., omeprazole, that inhibits CYP2C19 activity, metabolize clopidogrel poorly, have lower degrees of platelet inhibition (so-called "clopidogrel resistance"), and may be more likely to develop adverse cardiovascular events, especially stent thrombosis after ACS or PCI.

Newer ADP receptor blockers have been developed to address these shortcomings. *Prasugrel* (Effient) is an irreversible, oral thienopyridine with more rapid, potent, and consistent platelet inhibition than clopidogrel. In high risk ACS patients undergoing PCI (particularly those with diabetes or a drug eluting stent), prasugrel has been shown to further reduce ischemic events and stent thrombosis, but at a cost of increased risk of bleeding, particularly in patients who are older

(> 75 years), with low body weight (< 60 kg), and in those with a history of prior TIA or stroke (in whom the drug is contraindicated).

Ticagrelor (Brilinta) is the first reversible, oral nonthienopyridine ADP receptor blocker, in a new class called cyclopentyltriazolopyrimidine. Like prasugrel, it provides faster, greater, and more consistent platelet inhibition than clopidogrel, but with a more rapid "offset" of action. In ACS patients managed medically or with PCI, ticagrelor results in fewer vascular deaths, MIs, and stent thromboses than clopidogrel, without an increase in overall major bleeding, but with an increased rate of non-CABG related bleeding, and other adverse effects (e.g., dyspnea, ventricular pauses). Due to the faster recovery of platelet function, ticagrelor may be stopped 5 days before CABG or other surgery, rather than 7 days recommended for prasugel. Its twice-daily dosing and faster "offset" of antiplatelet effect, however, underscores the importance of patient compliance. Maintenance doses of aspirin above 100 mg daily may decrease the effectiveness of ticagrelor and should be avoided. Of note, *cangrelor* (Kengreal) is a potent, reversible IV nonthienopyridine ADP receptor blocker recently approved to reduce the risk of thrombotic events in ACS patients undergoing PCI who have not been pretreated with an oral P2Y12 platelet inhibitor. With its short half-life (3-6 minutes) and very rapid onset and offset of action, cangrelor may find a niche role for bridging off of other antiplatelet agents or as an alternative to GP IIb/IIIa receptor antagonists.

Thrombin Receptor (PAR-1) Antagonist

Vorapaxar (Zontivity), a first-in-class, selective, reversibly binding, oral thrombin receptor (PAR-1) platelet antagonist, has recently been approved as "add-on" therapy to aspirin and/or clopidogrel to reduce the risk of thrombotic cardiovascular events in select patients with prior MI or PAD. However, the increased risk of bleeding, particularly intracranial, precludes its use in patients with a history of stroke or TIA.

Glycoprotein IIb/IIIa Receptor Inhibitors (e.g., Abciximab, Eptifibatide, Tirofiban)

The most effective antiplatelet agents are the glycoprotein (GP) IIb/IIIa inhibitors. These agents reversibly inhibit the critical and final common pathway of platelet aggregation— the binding of activated GP IIb/IIIa receptors to fibrinogen and von Willebrand factor—and thus prevent platelets from sticking to one another, thereby impairing the formation of a hemostatic plug. (**Figure 12-1**) Intravenous GP IIb/IIIa inhibitors may be used in high-risk ACS patients (i.e., ST depression, elevated troponin levels), especially those with recurrent ischemia, a large thrombus burden, and/or inadequate pre-treatment with dual antiplatelet therapy at the time of PCI. These agents have been shown to reduce adverse cardiac events (e.g., MI, death). The currently approved agents include the small molecules *eptifiba-*

tide (Integrilin) and *tirofiban* (Aggrastat) for use in ACS, as well as the monoclonal antibody *abciximab* (ReoPro) for use in high-risk PCIs (e.g., patients with diabetes, chronic renal insufficiency, ST elevation MI). Recent studies in patients with acute ST elevation MI have demonstrated that intravenous GP IIb/IIIa inhibitors given in combination with a reduced dose of a thrombolytic agent reduces reinfarction, but does not confer a mortality benefit, and is associated with an increased risk of bleeding, particularly in the elderly. Rarely, an immune-mediated thrombocytopenia may also occur. Of note, oral GP IIb/IIIa inhibitors have been developed but have not demonstrated beneficial outcomes in clinical trials.

Chapter 13. Thrombolytics and Anticoagulants

Thrombolytic Agents (e.g., Streptokinase, Alteplase, Reteplase, Tenecteplase)

With rupture of a coronary artery atherosclerotic plaque, a platelet plug forms. In addition, the biochemical coagulation pathway may also be activated, resulting in a thrombus, containing not only platelets, but red blood cells and the reaction end products of the blood clotting processes, particularly fibrin. Once a thrombus has formed, the only clinically useful pharmacologic strategy involves degrading fibrin with thrombolytic therapy. Thrombolytic agents convert plasminogen to plasmin, thereby activating the endogenous fibrinolytic system and dissolving occlusive fibrin clots (**Figure 12-1**).

In the treatment of acute MI, thrombolytic therapy is aimed at rapid and complete restoration of coronary blood flow through the infarct-related artery; it is indicated for patients who present within 12 hours of the onset of chest pain with either ST segment elevation MI (where there is complete thrombotic coronary artery occlusion) or new (or presumably new) LBBB (suggesting an acute coronary thrombosis has taken place). The goal is to minimize "door-to-needle" time to less than 30 minutes. Early reperfusion reduces infarct size, preserves LV function, reduces the risk of arrhythmias, and improves survival.

Streptokinase (Streptase) is an older non-clot selective agent that stimulates the conversion of circulating plasminogen to plasmin, thus producing a systemic lytic response. *Alteplase* (tPA, Activase), along with the newer fibrin selective agents, *reteplase* (rPA, Retevase), and *tenecteplase* (TNK-tPA, TNKase) activate circulating plasminogen to a lesser extent than surface bound (intracoronary clot) plasminogen. All agents, however, activate circulating plasminogen to varying degrees and, as a result, bleeding is the most important risk of thrombolytic drugs. Since the major risk of thrombolysis is bleeding, contraindications to thrombolytics include patients with prior intracranial hemorrhage, known cerebrovascular lesion (e.g., neoplasm, aneurysm, AV malformation), active internal bleeding (excluding menses), suspected aortic dissection, recent ischemic stroke or significant closed head or facial trauma within 3 months. Thrombolytic agents have not been proven effective for non-ST segment elevation MI or unstable angina and, in fact, there is evidence that these agents may be harmful.

Recognition of the importance of coronary thrombosis in the pathogenesis of acute MI has led to the intensive development and application of the newer fibrinolytic agents (i.e., double bolus *reteplase* [rPA] and single bolus *tenecteplase*

[TNK-tPA] injection). These newer agents, both mutants of tPA with longer half lives, are currently favored over the "gold standard" tPA because of the ease of bolus administration vs. infusion. No thrombolytic agent is ideal for all patients, however, and each has its own advantages and disadvantages. Regardless of which agent is chosen, appropriate and prompt administration is the key to improving survival and quality of life. Specifics of the indications and precautions for the thrombolytic drugs are discussed in the approach to the patient with acute MI in Chapter 16.

Unfractionated and Low Molecular Weight Heparin, Direct Thrombin Inhibitors, and Factor Xa Inhibitors

Heparin anticoagulation (both IV *unfractionated heparin* [UFH] and subcutaneous *low molecular weight heparin* [LMWH] e.g., *enoxaparin* [Lovenox], *dalteparin* [Fragmin]) has also received renewed attention for the treatment of acute coronary syndromes. Heparin enhances the natural anticoagulant properties of antithrombin III, which prevents activation of the coagulation cascade (increases the rate of destruction of activated clotting factors II [thrombin], IX, X, XI, XII), and interferes with the ability of fibrinogen to form fibrin (**Figure 12-1**). Unfractionated heparin is administered parenterally as an intravenous bolus followed by a continuous infusion. Commercial preparations of IV unfractionated heparin are obtained from bovine or porcine sources. The adequacy of anticoagulation with unfractionated heparin can be determined by monitoring the activated partial thromboplastin time (aPTT) or the activated clotting time (ACT). Weight based protocols have become more popular in light of studies that have demonstrated their superiority over non-weight based treatment.

The most common clinical settings in which UFH is being used include unstable angina, non-STEMI, STEMI with PCI or fibrinolytic therapy (i.e., tPA, rPA, TNK-tPA), pulmonary embolism or deep vein thrombosis (DVT). When administering heparin, keep in mind additional drug-drug interactions. IV nitroglycerin may interfere with the anticoagulant effects of heparin. When using both these agents together, patients may require higher doses of IV heparin and should have their PTT levels monitored carefully. Discontinuation of nitroglycerin while heparin treatment is maintained may increase the risk of bleeding and thus require careful monitoring of PTT. Abrupt discontinuation of heparin therapy may result in a rebound effect.

The most important side effect of heparin is bleeding. Another potential adverse effect is immune-mediated, *heparin-induced thrombocytopenia* (HIT) (~3% of cases). HIT can lead to life-threatening bleeding, and has also been associated, paradoxically, with an increased risk of thrombosis (caused by antibodies directed against heparin-platelet complexes, resulting in platelet activation, aggregation, and clot production). The incidence of HIT may be reduced with porcine heparin compared to bovine heparin and with LMWH. Treatment of documented HIT includes discontinuation of all heparin products (SQ, IV, heparin flushes and heparin-coated catheters, as well as LMWH), and institution of alternative anti-coagulation i.e., *direct thrombin inhibitors*, that block both circulating and clot-bound thrombin, e.g., lepirudin (Refludan), a recombinant hirudin; argatroban, and bivalirudin (Angiomax), or *factor Xa inhibitors*, e.g., fondaparinux (Arixtra), that indirectly inhibit thrombin generation. Of note, IV bivalirudin is approved for use in patients with ACS undergoing PCI, and has been shown to reduce bleeding events, but at an increased risk (and cost) of acute stent thrombosis, when compared with heparin with or without GP IIb/IIIa inhibitors. Sub Q fondaparinux has been shown to be superior to UFH in patients with STEMI, and superior to LMWH in patients with non-ST elevation ACS, but with less bleeding. In patients undergoing PCI, however, UFH must be added since fondaparinux alone increases the risk of catheter thrombosis.

In addition to a lower risk of HIT, LMWH offers several other advantages over unfractionated heparin. LMWH has a long half life and can be easily administered SQ twice daily. It has greater anti-Xa activity than unfractionated heparin, resulting in a greater inhibition of thrombin generation. Due to its enhanced bio-availability and more reliable anticoagulation effect, there is no need for PTT measurements with LMWH. Furthermore, the use of LMWH is associated with similar or less bleeding than standard IV unfractionated heparin. LMWH is a suitable (may be preferable) alternative to unfractionated heparin in patients with unstable angina, non-ST/ST elevation MI, and in those undergoing PCI. Current clinical indications for LMWH also include prevention and/or treatment of deep vein thrombosis (DVT) (with or without pulmonary embolism). The use of LMWH, however, has not been adequately studied for thromboprophylaxis in patients with mechanical prosthetic heart valves. Cases of prosthetic heart valve thrombosis (including in pregnant women) have been reported.

Vitamin K Antagonists (e.g., Warfarin) and Novel Oral Anticoagulants (e.g., Dabigatran, Rivaroxaban, Apixaban, Edoxaban)

An increased risk of thromboembolism is associated with many common cardiac disorders, including atrial fibrillation (especially in patients >65 years of age, or those who have hypertension, a history of stroke or TIA, CHF, an LV ejection fraction < 40%, and diabetes mellitus), rheumatic mitral valve disease, acute MI (particularly anterior MI with LV dysfunction, LV aneurysm, and mural thrombus formation), and mechanical prosthetic heart valves. The long-term management, with oral anticoagulation therapy, of selective cardiac conditions associated with an increased risk of thromboembolism has resulted in a significant reduction in morbidity and mortality. The mainstay of oral anticoagulation therapy in patients with cardiovascular disease is *warfarin* (Coumadin), a vitamin K antagonist. Warfarin interferes with the formation of the reduced form of vitamin K, which is necessary in the activation of coagulation factors II (prothrombin), VII, IX, and X (**Figure 12-1**). The dose response differs significantly from patient to patient. Keep in mind that the half-life of factor VII (3–6 hours) is shorter than the half-life of factor II (~72 hours). Warfarin can elevate the prothrombin time (PT) before achieving a true antithrombotic state. Since warfarin's anticoagulation action has a delayed onset (2–7 days), unfractionated heparin or LMWH should be used concurrently at first (so-called "bridging") if an immediate effect is needed. Furthermore, because warfarin also impairs the function of certain vitamin K dependent natural coagulation inhibitors e.g., protein C (which also has a shorter half-life than factor II), theoretical concern exists regarding precipitating a hypercoagulable state before achieving a true antithrombotic state, if heparin-warfarin therapy is not overlapped. Warfarin's effect on coagulation must be monitored closely until individual doses are determined. Over the past several years, the international normalized ratio (INR), obtained by either venipuncture or by simple "finger-stick", has replaced the prothrombin time (PT) as the standard for monitoring oral anticoagulation. The desired therapeutic range for the INR in most cardiac conditions is 2–3. For patients with mechanical heart valves (particularly mitral), or those with higher risk characteristics, the INR should be 2.5–3.5. Of note, many experts recommend the addition of low dose aspirin to warfarin in patients with mechanical heart valves unless there is a contraindication. For select patients at increased risk of bleeding (e.g., those with coronary stents and atrial fibrillation), who require dual antiplatelet therapy and warfarin (so-called "triple therapy"), a low dose (81 mg) of aspirin (for a relatively short duration of time) along with clopidogrel and warfarin (with a target INR of 2.0-2.5), may be reasonable.

If your patient is on warfarin, many different drugs and/or foods can effect the INR levels, so caution should be exercised whenever new medications are administered, or dietary changes take place. (**Figure 13-1**). The safest rule is to tell your patient not to use any new or over the counter drugs (including herbal medicines) without first consulting with you. Commonly used herbal supplements include: Dong quai, Feverfew, Garlic, Ginger, Ginkgo Biloba, Glucosamine sulfate/chondroitin sulfate (which may increase risk of bleeding when combined with warfarin), Coenzyme Q10, Ginseng, and green tea (which may decrease risk of bleeding in patients on warfarin). Whenever these medications are started or stopped, more frequent monitoring of the PT/INR is necessary. Foods e.g., fish oil, mango, grapefruit juice, and cranberry juice, may raise the PT/INR, whereas high vitamin K containing green salads may lower the PT/INR level. Reduction of warfarin dose is required in the presence of decreased liver blood flow (CHF), liver damage (alcohol, malnutrition), or renal impairment.

Anticoagulation must be reversed for most types of surgery. However, minimally invasive procedures (e.g., dental cleaning) usually can be performed with the patient anticoagulated. Surgery generally can be done once the INR has fallen below 1.5. If the patient needs to remain on anticoagulation therapy as close to the time of surgery as possible, IV unfractionated heparin or SQ low molecular weight heparin, e.g., enoxaparin (Lovenox) can be started while the PT/INR is drifting down toward baseline, discontinued 6 hours prior to surgery, and resumed (usually without a bolus) ≥12 hours after surgery (in the absence of overt bleeding). In cases where the risk of thromboembolism is low (e.g., nonvalvular atrial fibrillation), warfarin may be discontinued several days before surgery and resumed

Figure 13-1

COMMONLY USED MEDICATIONS AND FOODS THAT AFFECT ANTICOAGULATION

INCREASES PT/INR	DECREASES PT/INR
Acetaminophen	Barbiturates
Allopurinol	Cholestyramine and colestipol
Amiodarone	Green leafy vegetables (e.g., broccoli, brussel sprouts, lettuce, spinach)— high vitamin K intake
Anabolic steroids Antibiotics (e.g., crythromycin, metronidazole, fluoroquinolones, trimethoprim-sulfa, 2nd and 3rd generation cephalosporins)	Herbal medicines (e.g., ginseng, St. John's Wort, Coenzyme Q10)
Cimetidine	Rifampin
Corticosteroids	Sucralfate
Fibrates	Vitamin C (high dose)
Heparin	
Herbal medicines (e.g., garlic, ginger, ginkgo, glucosamine)	
Isoniazid	
Nonsteroidal anti-inflammatory agents (including celecoxib [Celebrex], rofecoxib [Vioxx])	
Propafenone	
Quinidine	
Thyroxine	
Verapamil	
Vitamin E (high dose)	

shortly thereafter, without the use of perioperative heparin. The most common adverse effect of warfarin is bleeding. The risk of bleeding is directly related to the intensity and duration of therapy and may be increased by concomitant treatment with antiplatelet agents, age >65 years, and the use of medications that can elevate the PT/INR. If serious bleeding arises, warfarin's effect can be reversed within hours by the administration of Vitamin K, or even more quickly by transfusing fresh frozen plasma, which directly replenishes functional circulating clotting factors. Warfarin is teratogenic and should not be taken during pregnancy, especially in the first trimester.

Novel (non-vitamin K-dependent) oral anticoagulants (NOACs), e.g., the direct thrombin inhibitor, *dabigatran* (Pradaxa), and factor Xa inhibitors, *rivar-*

oxaban (Xarelto), *apixaban* (Eliquis) and *edoxaban* (Savaysa), produce reliable anticoagulation without the need for PT/INR monitoring, and are safe and effective alternatives to warfarin for the prevention of stroke and systemic embolism in patients with "nonvalvular" atrial fibrillation (i.e., without a mechanical valve or rheumatic MS), and the treatment of DVT and pulmonary embolism. In contrast to warfarin, NOACs can be given at fixed doses, have a rapid onset of action (that obviates the need for bridging therapy), fewer dietary and drug interactions, and less intracranial bleeding, but are more expensive. If serious bleeding occurs, specific antidotes, e.g., idarucizumab (Praxbind) for dabigatran, and andexanet alfa (Andexxa) for factor Xa inhibitors, are now approved for use to reverse their anticoagulation effect.

Chapter 14.   Lipid Controlling Agents

Serum lipids play an essential role in the pathogenesis of atherosclerosis. Lipid controlling drugs, particularly statins, can slow the rate of progression, improve clinical outcomes, and reduce mortality rates. Treatment strategies focus first on diet (low in saturated and trans fats, and if the patient is overweight, in total caloric intake) and exercise (which increases serum concentration of HDL). Drug therapy is generally reserved for patients who fail to respond to these lifestyle measures. Lipid controlling agents act on various aspects of lipid absorption and metabolism (**Figure 14-1**). Since these agents work by different mechanisms, they are sometimes combined to achieve a greater effect than possible by mono-drug therapy alone.

Figure 14-1. Lipid pathways and sites of drug intervention. (Modified from Goldberg, S. Clinical Physiology Made Ridiculously Simple). Exogenous pathway: Lipids in the diet are taken up by intestinal cells and formed into chylomicrons. Chylomicrons are released into the bloodstream and are hydrolyzed by lipoprotein lipase in fat and muscle cells. The action of lipoprotein lipase liberates triglycerides and releases chylomicron remnants. Chylomicron remnants are taken up by the liver and cleaved, resulting in free cholesterol. Endogenous pathway: The liver synthesizes very low density lipoproteins (VLDLs). VLDLs are released into the bloodstream and cleaved by lipoprotein lipase. This results in the liberation of triglycerides and intermediate density lipoproteins (IDLs). IDLs can either be taken up by low density lipoprotein (LDL)-receptors on the liver or further hydrolyzed to release triglycerides and form LDLs. LDLs bind to their receptors on extrahepatic or hepatic tissues. HDLs are formed by peripheral cells and serve to transport cholesterol to the liver. The effects of drug therapy can be understood from these pathways. *Statins* inhibit the HMG Co-A reductase enzyme and decrease the synthesis of cholesterol and secretion of VLDL, and increase the activity of LDL receptors. *Bile acid binding resins* increase the secretion of bile acids (along with cholesterol). *Niacin* increases the secretion of VLDL and the formation of LDL and increases the formation of HDL. *Fibrates* decrease the secretion VLDL and increase the activity of lipoprotein lipase, thereby increasing the removal of triglycerides. *Ezetimibe* inhibits the intestinal absorption of cholesterol (both from the diet and via enterohepatic reabsorption), and lowers LDL cholesterol. *PCSK9 inhibitors* block the degradation of hepatic LDL receptors, which in turn increases the clearance of LDL cholesterol from the blood. Of note, lipoprotein (a) [Lp (a)], a genetic variant of LDL, is synthesized and secreted primarily by the liver, but the receptors that bind and mediate its catabolism are not well understood.

Figure 14-1

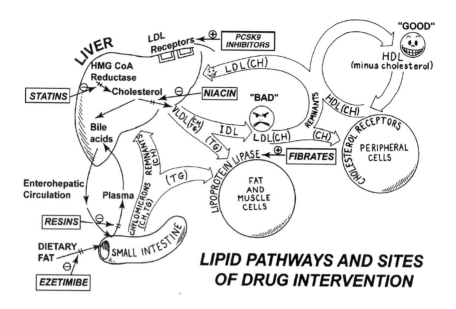

LIPID PATHWAYS AND SITES OF DRUG INTERVENTION

The most commonly used drugs used in the treatment of dyslipidemia include the following:

HMG-CoA Reductase Inhibitors ("Statins")

"Statins" e.g., *lovastatin* (Mevacor), *pravastatin* (Pravachol), *simvastatin* (Zocor), *atorvastatin* (Lipitor), *fluvastatin* (Lescol), *rosuvastatin* (Crestor), and *pitavastatin* (Livalo) inhibit the enzyme HMG CoA reductase, a key rate-limiting component in the biochemical pathway for the synthesis of cholesterol. Inhibition of this pathway results in increased synthesis of LDL receptors, which lowers serum cholesterol. They are highly effective in reducing "bad" LDL cholesterol ($\downarrow$ 18–55%) and moderately effective in raising "good" HDL cholesterol ($\uparrow$ 5–15%) and in reducing triglyceride levels ($\downarrow$ 7–30%). The benefits of statin therapy may extend beyond lipid-lowering. These agents can potentially improve endothelial dysfunction, inhibit platelet aggregation, impair thrombus formation, and reduce inflammation and thus "stabilize" atherosclerotic plaques, which makes them less prone to rupture and consequently reduces clinical CAD events and mortality. They are generally well tolerated but may occasionally raise liver enzymes and blood sugar levels, can cause headache, fatigue, memory loss, constipation, flatulence, dyspepsia, and abdominal pain, and rarely skeletal muscle damage (muscle pain, tenderness or weakness), particularly if used in high doses or when combined with niacin or a fibrate (especially gemfibrozil). Blood tests, e.g., liver function tests (LFTs), creatine kinase (CK), should be obtained initially and when clinically indicated thereafter, to determine whether statins need to be discontinued (**Note:** If LFTs > 3 times and/or CK ≥10 times the upper limit of normal, stop statin therapy). Although risk for muscle toxicity exists with all statins, concern has been raised about a potentially greater risk with high dose simvastatin.

Nicotinic Acid (Niacin)

Niacin reduces the production of the triglyceride-containing very low density lipoproteins (VLDLs) in the liver, which in turn, lowers serum LDL cholesterol levels. It is inexpensive and effective in lowering LDL cholesterol ($\downarrow$ 5–25%), and particularly at raising HDL cholesterol ($\uparrow$ 15–35%) and lowering Lp(a), an LDL-like lipoprotein that carries an independent risk of ASCVD, by up to 30-40% (but the clinical benefit is uncertain), and triglyceride levels ($\downarrow$ 20–50%). Compliance can be a problem, however, because of flushing and prominent side effects, e.g., headache, itching, GI upset (do not use in patients with peptic ulcer), liver function abnormalities, increased glucose and uric acid levels. Taking aspirin a half hour before the niacin dose can help ameliorate the flushing reaction. Side effects are better tolerated with extended release preparations. Niaspan is a more recent extended-release form of niacin that has less hepatic toxicity and flushing than former controlled-release forms.

Bile Acid Sequestrants (Resins)

Bile acid sequestrants, e.g., *cholestyramine* (Questran), *colestipol* (Colestid), *colesevelam* (Welchol), are anion exchange resins that bind bile acids in the intestinal lumen, thereby promoting their loss from the GI tract. The resultant interruption of the enterohepatic circulation of bile acids promotes the conversion of cholesterol to bile acids in the liver. Reducing hepatic cholesterol content stimulates the formation of LDL receptors, which reduces serum cholesterol levels. Bile acid sequestrants are used mainly to treat high LDL cholesterol. These agents lower LDL cholesterol ($\downarrow$ 15–30%) but either do not change or increase triglyceride levels, and have only a minimal effect at raising HDL cholesterol ($\uparrow$ 3–5%). They are especially useful in combination with "statins". Resins may cause constipation, flatulence, nausea, heartburn, and can decrease the absorption of other medications (e.g., warfarin, digitalis).

Fibric Acid Derivatives

The fibric acid derivatives e.g., *gemfibrozil* (Lopid), *fenofibrate* (Tricor), *fenofibric acid* (Trilipix), increase the activity of the enzyme lipoprotein lipase, which enhances catabolism of triglyceride-rich VLDLs and IDLs, and reduces serum triglyceride levels. These agents lower high triglyceride levels ($\downarrow$ 20–50%) more effectively than high LDL cholesterol levels ($\downarrow$ 5–20%) and increase HDL cholesterol ($\uparrow$ 10–20%). They are generally well tolerated but may cause GI upset (nausea, abdominal pain), cholelithiasis, worsen renal insufficiency, potentiate the effects of warfarin, and can cause myositis or rhabdomyolysis when used alone or in combination with a "statin". Consider fibrates or niacin if HDL cholesterol level is low or triglyceride level is high. Reduction in elevated triglyceride levels can decrease the risk of pancreatitis.

Cholesterol Absorption Inhibitors (e.g., Ezetimibe)

Ezetimibe (Zetia), a *cholesterol absorption inhibitor*, which prevents dietary and biliary cholesterol from crossing the intestinal wall and getting into the blood stream, reduces LDL cholesterol ($\downarrow$ 18–25%), increases HDL cholesterol ($\uparrow$ 1–3%) and reduces triglyceride levels ($\downarrow$ 8–14%). The drug is generally well tolerated, but may raise liver enzymes, particularly when combined with a statin, and on rare occasion has been associated with myalgias, rhabdomyolysis, acute pancreatitis, and thrombocytopenia. Ezetimibe may be an additional drug to consider if the LDL cholesterol level remains high despite the maximum recommended and/or tolerated dose of statin. Recent data has shown that the addition of ezetimibe to a statin in high risk ACS patients further reduces cardiovascular events when compared to statin therapy alone.

Proprotein Convertase Subtilisin-Kexin Type 9 (PCSK9) Inhibitors

Injectable monoclonal antibodies, e.g., *alirocumab* (Praluent) and *evolocumab* (Repatha) that inhibit the function of proprotein convertase subtilisin-kexin type 9, so-called *PCSK9 inhibitors*, block the degradation of hepatic LDL receptors, which in turn increases LDL cholesterol clearance, and reduces serum LDL cholesterol levels ($\downarrow$ 40-70%). These agents have been approved as an adjunct to statin therapy for high risk patients with familial hypercholesterolemia or known ASCVD, and may become suitable alternative therapy for patients who are statin-intolerant.

Chapter 15. Antiarrhythmic Agents

The pharmacologic treatment of patients with cardiac arrhythmias requires substantial knowledge about the rhythm disorder and antiarrhythmic drugs. It is necessary to choose the effective drug that is least likely to harm the patient. The major factors to be considered include side effects, the presence and severity of LV dysfunction, hepatic and renal insufficiency, and the drug profile. (**Figure 15-1**). The most common classification of drugs used for the treatment of cardiac arrhythmias (based on their electrophysiologic actions) is the modified *Vaughan-Williams classification*. This system includes:

- Classes IA, B and C (*sodium channel blockers*)
- Class II (*beta-receptor blockers*)
- Class III (*potassium channel blockers*) and
- Class IV (*calcium channel blockers*)

An understanding of the mechanism by which action potentials are propagated through conducting cells facilitates learning about the mechanism of antiarrhythmic action (**Figure 15-2**).

Figure 15-2. Left. Relationship of the phases (0–4) of a cardiac action potential from a Purkinje fiber (top) to the cardiac electrical activity on the surface ECG (bottom). Top. Phase 0: Voltage-dependent Na^+ channels open and a rapid movement of sodium ions inward stimulates (depolarizes) the cell. Phase 1: Early phase of repolarization, caused by inactivation of Na^+ influx and the activation of a transient outward K^+ current. Phase 2: Plateau phase, characterized by low membrane conductance and the activation of a slow inward Ca^{++} current (and relatively low K^+ efflux). Phase 3: Rapid repolarization to resting potential results from outward K^+ current. Phase 4 (diastole): Outward K^+ current is deactivated and an inward Na^+ current reduces transmembrane potential. In normal ventricular muscle cells, the resting potential during phase 4 remains in the region of −80 to −90 mV. Bottom. Phase 0 depolarization is reflected in the QRS complex on the ECG. The repolarization period (phases 2 and 3) constitutes the action potential duration that governs the refractory period of heart muscle, and is represented on the surface ECG by the QT interval. **Right.** Sinus node action potential. Not all cells in the cardiac conduction system rely on sodium influx for initial depolarization. In sinus node (shown here) and AV nodal cells, spontaneous diastolic (phase 4) depolarization is mediated primarily by a slow inward movement of calcium ions and, to a lesser extent, sodium ions (I_f "funny" current).

Figure 15-1

ANTIARRHYTHMIC DRUG THERAPY

VAUGHAN-WILLIAMS DRUG CLASSIFICATION	CLINICAL INDICATIONS	SIDE EFFECTS
Class I A Quinidine (Quinidex)	Conversion/prevention of atrial fibrillation, atrial flutter, ventricular tachycardia.	Diarrhea, proarrhythmia ($\uparrow$ QT, torsades de pointes), thrombocytopenia, 1:1 flutter (vagolytic effect), rash, cinchonism (tinnitus, hearing loss)
Procainamide (Procan)	Prevention of ventricular fibrillation.	Nausea, lupus-like syndrome, drug fever, agranulocytosis, proarrhythmia ($\uparrow$ QT, torsades de pointes), 1:1 flutter (vagolytic effect)
Disopyramide (Norpace)		Myocardial depression, proarrhythmia ($\uparrow$ QT, torsades de pointes), 1:1 flutter, anticholinergic effects (urinary retention, dry mouth, blurred vision, constipation)
Class I B Lidocaine (Xylocaine) Mexiletine (Mexitil)	Treatment of ventricular tachyarrhythmias	Drowsiness, slurred speech, confusion, seizures, respiratory arrest. Nausea, tremor, gait disturbance
Class I C Flecainide (Tambocor) Propafenone (Rythmol)	Conversion/prevention of atrial fibrillation, atrial flutter, ventricular tachycardia. Prevention of ventricular fibrillation.	CNS, visual, and GI disturbances, VT (proarrhythmia), 1:1 flutter, CHF Metallic taste; CNS, visual, and GI disturbances, VT (proarrhythmia), CHF, increases serum digoxin and INR (warfarin) levels
Class II β-blockers	Rate control for atrial fibrillation, atrial flutter; prevention of supraventricular tachycardia, with adjunctive ventricular antiarrhythmic therapy.	Marked bradycardia, AV block, bronchospasm, fatigue, depression, cold hands and feet, vivid dreams, memory loss, impotence. May worsen CHF and diabetic control.

49

Figure 15-1

ANTIARRHYTHMIC DRUG THERAPY (Continued)

VAUGHAN-WILLIAMS DRUGCLASSIFICATION	CLINICAL INDICATIONS	SIDE EFFECTS
Class III Amiodarone (Cordarone)	Conversion/prevention of atrial fibrillation, atrial flutter, ventricular tachycardia.	Thyroid abnormalities, pulmonary fibrosis, hepatitis, corneal microdeposits, bluish-gray skin discoloration, neuropathy, ↑ QT, increased sensitivity to warfarin.
Sotalol (Betapace)	Prevention of atrial and ventricular fibrillation.	Fatigue, bradycardia, exacerbation of ventricular arrhythmia, ↑ QT, torsades de pointes
Ibutilide (Corvert)	Conversion of atrial fibrillation/flutter	Torsades de pointes, hypotension, nausea
Dofetilide (Tikosyn)	Conversion/prevention of atrial fibrillation/flutter	↑ QT, torsades de pointes, headache, dizziness
Dronedarone (Multaq)	Prevention of atrial fibrillation/flutter	Nausea, vomiting, diarrhea, abdominal pain, asthenia, ↑ QT
Class IV Calcium channel blockers Verapamil (Calan, Isoptin), Diltiazem (Cardizem)	Rate control for atrial fibrillation/flutter, conversion of SVT	Bradycardia, AV block, edema, may worsen CHF, hypotension, constipation (verapamil).
Other Agents Digoxin (Lanoxin)	Rate control for atrial fibrillation/flutter	GI and visual disturbances, AV block, ventricular and supraventricular arrhythmias
Adenosine (Adenocard)	Conversion of SVT	Facial flushing, chest pain, dyspnea, transient hypo-tension and/or atrial standstill (lasting <10 seconds)

Antiarrhythmic drugs influence cardiac conduction properties (usually by modifying ion conductance) and may revert an abnormal rhythm to normal sinus rhythm. They work primarily by reducing ectopic pacemaker activity and/or altering conduction in reentrant circuits. Each class of antiarrhythmic drugs acts on a different phase of the action potential. Class I agents (sodium channel blockers) decrease the upstroke velocity during phase 0 of the action potential. Class II agents (beta blockers) inhibit phase 4 spontaneous depolarization (and indirectly close calcium channels). Class III agents (potassium channel blockers) block the outward potassium channel during phase 3 and prolong the action potential duration and refractoriness (resistance to stimulation). Class IV agents (the rate slowing calcium channel blockers [i.e., verapamil and diltiazem]) inhibit the influx of calcium, which is most responsible for pacemaker automaticity and conduction in the sinus and AV nodes.

Although the electrophysiological effects of most of the antiarrhythmic agents have been defined, their use in controlling arrhythmias remains largely empirical. They must be used carefully since in certain settings they can exacerbate arrhythmias ("proarrhythmic effect"), and most can depress LV function. They should be used with caution, if at all, for patients with life-threatening ventricular arrhythmias and symptomatic SVTs. The following points are of practical use to the clinician and deserve special mention.

Class I Agents

Classes I A, B, and C antiarrhythmic drugs predominately slow the maximum velocity of the upstroke of the Purkinje fiber action potential (phase 0) by blocking the influx of sodium ions into the cell (which decreases the rate of depolarization). (**Figure 15-2**). In clinical trials, these agents have not been shown to decrease mortality in many subsets of patients at risk for sudden cardiac death. In fact, they have been shown to increase mortality (proarrhythmic effect) in certain subsets of patients with structural heart disease (particularly those with the most advanced LV dysfunction) and to have no effect on the mortality of others. There is evidence, however, that beta blockers reduce mortality rate, especially in patients with CAD and CHF. In patients who have survived a cardiac arrest or who present with symptomatic VT/VF, guided therapy with group I drugs is inferior to guided therapy with sotalol (Betapace, a Class III antiarrhythmic agent with both Class II beta blocker properties and Class III activity), empiric treatment with amiodarone (Cordarone, a Class III drug), or therapy with an ICD. The use of class I drugs is increasingly being relegated to patients who have symptomatic arrhythmias with no demonstrable structural heart disease. Although proarrhythmic effects may occur in these patients, they are not usually fatal.

51

Figure 15-2

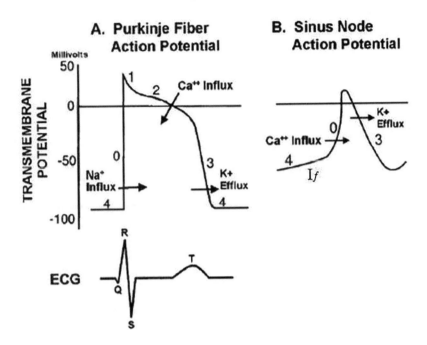

Class IA Agents (e.g., Quinidine, Procainamide, Disopyramide) (Figure 15-1)

Class IA agents moderately slow the rate of rise of the Purkinje fiber action potential and prolong its duration, thus slowing conduction, prolonging repolarization, and increasing refractoriness. These agents particularly affect Purkinje fibers and ectopic pacemakers. These actions can prolong the QRS and QT intervals on the surface ECG. Class IA agents are effective at converting and suppressing a variety of reentrant and ectopic SVTs (e.g., atrial fibrillation and flutter, paroxysmal SVT) as well as suppressing ventricular ectopy (however, they are associated with significantly increased mortality, when used in patients who have structural heart disease). When given to a patient with atrial fibrillation or flutter, class IA agents may increase the ventricular response rate as the atrial rate slows since these agents can also enhance conduction through the AV node by means of their vagolytic effects. A drug with AV nodal blocking properties (e.g., digoxin, beta blockers, verapamil, diltiazem) should be given first. Since *quinidine* (sulfate and gluconate) increases serum digoxin levels, the maintenance dose of digoxin will have to be decreased.

Procainamide (Procan, Pronestyl) is more commonly used in the acute management of arrhythmias. Hypotension may result with rapid IV loading doses.

Sixty to seventy percent of patients who receive procainamide develop antinuclear antibodies. Long-term use is associated with a clinical lupus-like syndrome in ~30% of patients (reversible on stopping the drug).

Disopyramide (Norpace) has prominent anticholinergic effects (especially urinary retention, dry mouth, blurred vision, constipation, aggravation of narrow angle glaucoma) and may worsen established heart failure. Disopyramide has significant negative inotropic properties (i.e., decreases ventricular contractility) and should be used with extreme caution (if at all) in patients with LV systolic dysfunction. Class IA agents present a risk of cardiovascular mortality (proarrhythmic effect—"torsades de pointes"). As a result, use of the entire class IA drugs is gradually shifting to other agents (e.g., class III drugs) or devices for chronic use.

Class IB Agents (e.g., Lidocaine, Mexiletine, Tocainide, Phenytoin) (Figure 15-1)

Class IB agents mildly slow the rate of rise of the Purkinje fiber action potential and decrease its duration, shorten refractory period and repolarization, and slow conduction velocity through ischemic myocardium (suppresses ventricular automaticity). These agents cause no QRS or QT interval changes, so there is less risk of inducing a proarrhythmia than Class 1A drugs. IV *Lidocaine* (Xylocaine) is recommended for the treatment of symptomatic or life-threatening ventricular arrhythmias. Its primary use is for ischemic-related ventricular arrhythmias in the acute phase of an MI. Prophylactic lidocaine, however, is no longer recommended in the management of acute MI. In fact, it may be detrimental (increased mortality) in this setting. The loading and maintenance dose of lidocaine should be reduced in patients who metabolize the drug slowly (e.g., those with CHF, liver dysfunction, and in those >70 years of age). Toxicity is manifest primarily as central nervous system alterations ranging from tremor and lightheadedness to confusion, stupor, coma, and seizures.

Mexiletine (Mexitil) can be given orally for serious ventricular arrhythmias. As a single agent, potency is low and it is frequently combined with other antiarrhythmics.

Phenytoin (Dilantin), an anticonvulsant drug used extensively for the treatment of epilepsy, is particularly effective in treating atrial and ventricular arrhythmias caused by digitalis toxicity.

Class IC Agents (e.g., Propafenone, Flecainide, Encainide) (Figure 15-1)

Class IC agents markedly slow the upstroke rate of the Purkinje fiber action potential. They cause such a dramatic slowing of conduction in all cardiac tissues, thereby prolonging the PR and QRS intervals. The QT interval will be affected primarily because of QRS prolongation and not a repolarization effect (because these drugs do not profoundly influence repolarization). Class IC agents are effective in suppressing ventricular arrhythmias, but have a high proarrhythmic potential, particularly in the setting of CAD. Patients at highest risk for proarrhythmia have a history of MI or a low ejection fraction. When administered to post-MI patients with asymptomatic ventricular arrhythmias, flecainide and encainide (and moricizine, a class IA agent) were associated with an increase in mortality (when compared to placebo).

Both *flecainide* (Tambocor) and *propafenone* (Rythmol) have been shown to be effective in preventing recurrent episodes of paroxysmal atrial fibrillation and AV nodal reentrant tachyarrhythmias. Flecainide remains an effective and relatively safe therapy for SVTs (especially paroxysmal atrial fibrillation) in patients with structurally normal hearts and should be used, therefore, only in patients without underlying heart disease. Reports of atrial proarrhythmia include conversion of atrial fibrillation or flutter to flutter with 1:1 conduction. Propafenone is similar to flecainide but with weak beta blocking effects and therefore may exacerbate bradycardia, heart block, CHF, and bronchospasm. Propafenone should be administered with caution, therefore, in patients receiving beta blockers. Propafenone can also increase the serum level of digoxin and the INR with oral anticoagulants (warfarin).

Class II Agents (i.e., Beta Blockers, e.g., Propranolol, Metoprolol, Atenolol)

Class II agents are beta blockers. These drugs inhibit sympathetic nervous system stimulation of cardiac tissue by depressing phase 4 depolarization, thereby decreasing sinoatrial (SA) node automaticity and prolonging atrioventricular (AV) conduction. They prolong the PR interval on the ECG but have little (slightly shorten) or no effect on the QT interval. Beta blockers may be effective in slowing the ventricular response rate in atrial fibrillation or flutter, suppressing episodes of paroxysmal atrial fibrillation, converting paroxysmal reentrant SVTs, suppressing ventricular arrhythmias, preventing post-MI sudden death, suppressing MVP or catecholamine-induced ventricular ectopy, and minimizing QT-related "torsades de pointes" VT (since beta blockers do not prolong the QT interval). They have been shown to reduce the incidence of sudden death in a variety of patient populations and should, therefore, be considered in the therapy of patients with malignant VTs, especially in the setting of LV dysfunction or CAD.

Intravenous *esmolol* (Brevibloc) is useful, in view of its short half-life (~9 minutes) in patients at risk for the common complications of beta blockade (e.g., bradycardia, hypotension) Beta blockers as a class consistently reduce mortality (both total and sudden death). The increased prevalence of hypertension and CAD in patients with recurrent arrhythmias encourages the use of beta blockade for combined antiarrhythmic, antihypertensive, and antiischemic actions. Their long term proven safety and efficacy makes these agents the best initial choice for primary or adjunctive treatment of patients with supraventricular and ventricular arrhythmias.

Class III Agents (e.g., Sotalol, Amiodarone, Bretylium, Ibutilide, Dofetilide, Dronedarone)

Class III agents exert their antiarrhythmic effects primarily by blocking potassium channels during phase 3 of the action potential. They increase the action potential duration, prolong repolarization and refractoriness, widen the QRS complex, and prolong the QT interval. These agents decrease automaticity and conduction. All Class III antiarrhythmic drugs have proarrhythmic potential.

Sotalol (Betapace) is a non-selective beta blocker that also has Class III properties. It prolongs the QT interval (and therefore may precipitate torsades de pointes). Sotalol has been shown to be effective in the management of ventricular arrhythmias (superior to class I agents) and in the prevention and treatment of atrial fibrillation, but should be used with caution in patients with impaired LV function, as well as reduced renal function. It should not be initiated as an outpatient, if underlying structural heart disease is present.

Amiodarone (Cordarone) is an effective therapy for a wide range of supraventricular and ventricular arrhythmias, including atrial fibrillation and flutter, VT, and SVTs (including those involving bypass tracts). It is recommended as a first line agent for the prevention or treatment of atrial fibrillation in patients with CHF and has been shown to be more effective than class IA agents for the treatment of ventricular arrhythmias. In addition, amiodarone may decrease arrhythmic death after MI, but in patients with moderate to severe ischemic or nonischemic systolic CHF, long term use does not improve survival and may even be detrimental. Amiodarone may be administered IV for the acute treatment of hemodynamically significant and refractory life-threatening ventricular tachyarrhythmias, and is a first line drug for the emergency treatment of VT/VF during cardiac resuscitation. IV use may cause hypotension. When administered orally, it exerts a powerful suppressant effect on PVCs and non-sustained VT, and provides control in 60% to 80% of patients with recurrent VT/VF in whom conventional drugs have failed. However, serious adverse side effects, e.g., pulmonary fibrosis (rarely but occasionally irreversible), thyroid dysfunction, elevated liver enzymes, ataxia, peripheral neuropathy, as well as photosensitivity, blue-gray skin discoloration, corneal microdeposits may occur. Because of the multiple toxicities, patients taking amiodarone should undergo chest x-ray (CXR) examination and pulmonary function testing (to look for pulmonary fibrosis), liver function tests (to screen for hepatitis), and thyroid function studies (to check for hypo-or hyperthyroidism) every 6 months, along with a slit-lamp ophthalmic examination yearly (to look for corneal microdeposits). Low doses have demonstrated a major decline in the overall incidence of serious adverse reactions, and have been shown to be effective in suppressing SVTs, converting paroxysmal atrial fibrillation, and maintaining normal sinus rhythm after conversion. It has also recently been shown to be effective when administered IV to suppress sustained VT and prevent recurrent VF. QT prolongation is mild with only rare incidence of proarrhythmic "torsades de pointes". Amiodarone is contraindicated in patients with marked sinus bradycardia and second or third degree heart block in the absence of a functioning pacemaker. During long-term therapy, there is no impairment of LV function. Keep in mind that the drug has a long half-life (averaging 25–60 days) and therefore it takes a long time for the drug to reach therapeutic levels and to be cleared by the body. Amiodarone can increase the serum level of digoxin by 70% and the INR with oral anticoagulants (warfarin) by 100%.

IV *bretylium* has been used mainly in the past in the acute treatment of life-threatening ventricular arrhythmias unresponsive to other agents. Because of limited data to support its use, however, bretylium has been removed from the advanced cardiac life support (ACLS) list of antiarrhythmic agents for patients with pulseless VT or VF.

IV *ibutilide* (Corvert) is a parenteral class III agent approved for the rapid conversion of recent onset atrial fibrillation or flutter. Its role in clinical practice continues to evolve. It restores normal sinus rhythm in ~60–70% of patients with recent-onset atrial flutter and ~35–50% of patients with recent-onset atrial fibrillation and also enhances the success of electrical cardioversion. When effective, acute conversion occurs in the first hour after administration. Prolongation of the QT interval along with torsades de pointes may occur in 5–10% of cases. The reported proarrhythmic effects of IV ibutilide generally occur in the first 4 hours after termination of the IV infusion. Patients treated with ibutilide (and other antiarrhythmic agents that prolong the QT interval) should undergo continuous telemetry monitoring to follow for QT prolongation and the development of torsades de pointes.

Dofetilide (Tikosyn) is a recently approved oral class III antiarrhythmic drug that shows promise as a safe and effective treatment in patients with atrial fibrillation or flutter for inducing a reversion to normal sinus rhythm and maintaining sinus rhythm once it has been achieved. Similar to other class III agents (other than amiodarone), dofetilide's major adverse effect is QT prolongation complicated by torsades de pointes in a small percentage of patients. Therefore, its administration must be performed in the hospital during careful electrocardiographic monitoring.

Another class III agent recently approved is *dronedarone* (Multaq), a deiodinated analog of amiodarone with a much shorter half life (1 to 2 days vs. months) and the potential for less thyroid and pulmonary toxicity. Clinical trial data show a reduced risk of cardiovascular related hospitalization, along with rhythm and rate control, in hemodynamically stable patients treated for atrial fibrillation. Because of an increase in mortality, however, dronedarone is contraindicated in patients with permanent atrial fibrillation and advanced or recently decompensated CHF. Common adverse side effects include nausea, vomiting, diarrhea, and abdominal pain. Similar to amiodarone, dronedarone is rarely associated with torsades de pointes. However, dronedarone is substantially less effective than amiodarone in maintaining sinus rhythm. Patients taking dronedarone should undergo periodic liver function testing, since case reports of rare, but severe liver toxicity have emerged in association with its use.

Class IV Agents (i.e., Calcium Channel Blockers e.g., Verapamil, Diltiazem)

Class IV agents e.g., verapamil and diltiazem, are the slow calcium channel blockers. They are most potent in tissues in which the action potential depends on calcium currents, e.g., the SA and AV node. Within nodal tissue, rate slowing calcium channel blockers decrease SA node automaticity and prolong AV conduction and refractoriness. The ECG may show a prolonged PR interval or slowing of the sinus rate. These agents are useful in the treatment of reentry rhythms involving the AV node, and for slowing the ventricular response to atrial fibrillation and atrial flutter. IV verapamil and diltiazem, therefore, are effective in terminating paroxysmal reentrant SVTs and controlling the rapid ventricular response rate in atrial fibrillation or flutter. IV use can be complicated by hypotension and bradycardia (particularly in patients receiving beta blockers). Chronic oral therapy may be useful in preventing SVTs.

Diltiazem (Cardizem) can be used in conjunction with digoxin for rate control of atrial fibrillation. It is important to note, however, that *verapamil* (Calan, Isoptin) may raise digoxin levels. Beta blockers and rate-slowing calcium channel blockers, by virtue of their ability to selectively slow conduction in the AV node, may increase conduction down a bypass tract, and therefore, are contraindicated in patients with Wolff-Parkinson-White (WPW) syndrome. The dihydropyridine calcium channel blockers (e.g., nifedipine and amlodipine) do not cause electrophysiologic changes and are not used as antiarrhythmics. They are used primarily to treat patients with hypertension and CAD, including stable, unstable, or variant angina.

OTHER AGENTS

All antiarrhythmic drugs do not fit neatly into the above four classifications. As previously mentioned, sotalol possesses characteristics of both Class II and Class III drugs. Some drugs used to treat arrhythmias (e.g., digitalis, adenosine) do not fit into the classification system at all.

Digitalis

Digitalis, a cardiac glycoside, inhibits the Na^+/K^+-ATPase pump that maintains the sodium/potassium transmembrane gradients. It increases cardiac contractility and prolongs the refractory period of the AV node. Digitalis has visible effects on the ECG, i.e. coving or valley-like ST segment depression. Digitalis holds a firm place in the treatment of rapid atrial fibrillation and flutter by slowing conduction in the AV node. It is useful for controlling the ventricular response to an SVT and may also be effective in treating AV nodal and AV reentrant tachyarrhythmia. *Digoxin* (Lanoxin) is the drug of choice for rate control in the setting of CHF.

Effects of IV digoxin are delayed for 6 to 12 hours; therefore, IV calcium channel blockers or beta blockers are preferred for immediate rate control. Digoxin has minimal efficacy in the presence of high circulating catecholamines (e.g., during exercise or acute illness). Cardiac effects of digitalis toxicity include SA and AV blocks and junctional and ventricular arrhythmias.

Adenosine

Adenosine (Adenocard), a naturally occurring nucleoside that activates potassium channels, has substantial electrophysiologic effects on the sinus and AV nodes. This agent acts on the AV node to slow conduction and inhibit reentry pathways. It can be administered rapid IV bolus to terminate AV nodal or AV reentrant tachycardia (but is not effective in atrial fibrillation or flutter) in ~95% of cases. Transient side effects are common, including sinus bradycardia, AV block, flushing, chest pain, and dyspnea. Metabolism is very rapid with a half-life of 2 to 6 seconds, and adverse effects wear off within 1 minute. The drug should be used cautiously in patients with asthma or those receiving dipyridamole (Persantine). Higher doses may be needed if the patient is on theophylline or caffeine (since these methylxanthines competitively antagonize the adenosine receptor), and lower doses if the patient is on dipyridamole (since dipyridamole inhibits the breakdown of adenosine and enhances its effect).

Ivabradine

Ivabradine (Corlanor), is a novel agent that acts by selectively blocking the hyperpolarization-activated cyclic nucleotide-gated (HCN) channel, thereby inhibiting the inward Na^+/K^+ "funny current" (I_f) in the sinoatrial node, resulting in a dose dependent reduction in heart rate. The drug is approved for use as add-on therapy to reduce the risk of hospitalization (but not mortality) for worsening heart failure in patients with stable, symptomatic chronic heart failure with a reduced ejection fraction $\leq 35\%$, who are in sinus rhythm with a resting heart rate ≥ 70 beats per minute, and who are on maximum tolerated doses of beta blockers or have a contraindication to their use. Unlike beta blockers, ivabradine has no effect on myocardial contractility (no negative inotropic effect). Side effects include bradycardia, atrial fibrillation, and visual disturbances, called phosphenes (flashes of light), which are generally mild and resolve spontaneously. Ivabradine should not be used in combination with agents that prolong the QT interval and must be used cautiously with inhibitors (including grapefruit juice) or inducers of CYP3A4.

PART III.   APPROACH TO SPECIFIC CARDIOVASCULAR CONDITIONS

The previous chapters in this book provided practical, useful information on the vast array of cardiac drugs available in cardiology today. The following chapters "put it all together," and will provide contemporary practitioners and trainees with an up-to-date, "evidence-based" approach to the pharmacologic management of a broad spectrum of cardiovascular conditions that can easily be used to guide therapeutic decision-making in clinical practice. Where appropriate, current indications for the latest cardiac devices, interventional and surgical techniques will also be discussed.

Chapter 16.   Coronary Artery Disease

CAD represents, by far, the most common cardiac problem encountered in clinical practice today. It affects about 16 million Americans and remains the single leading cause of death in the United States. Annually, there are more than 5 million emergency department visits for evaluation of chest discomfort suggestive of an *acute coronary syndrome* (unstable angina, myocardial infarction). Over 1 million Americans experience a new or recurrent *myocardial infarction* (MI) each year. Many more are hospitalized for *unstable angina* and the evaluation and treatment of stable chest pain syndromes. In many cases of acute MI, death occurs early due to VF even before the patient has the opportunity to benefit from current catheter-based PCI and/or thrombolytic reperfusion therapy.

Figure 16-1. The clinical manifestations of CAD comprise a spectrum ranging from asymptomatic to sudden death.

In *stable angina*, the symptoms may arise from increased oxygen demand (*exertional angina*, resulting from flow-limiting coronary stenosis), or may follow coronary artery spasm (*variant angina*, also called *Prinzmetal's angina*), or a combination of stenosis and spasm. In *unstable angina*, the pathology is more ominous, involving plaque rupture or erosion with superimposed thrombus formation, which, if persistent, may result in a *myocardial infarction*. Patients with these *acute coronary syndromes* are at risk for *sudden death*.

Figure 16-1

CLINICAL SPECTRUM OF CORONARY ARTERY DISEASE

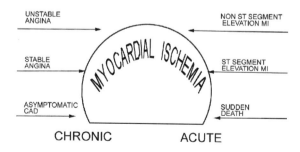

61

Figure 16-2. Pathophysiology of *acute coronary syndromes (ACS):* Endothelial dysfunction, inflammation, and formation of fatty streaks contribute to the development of an atherosclerotic plaque. Most ACS result from coronary thrombus formation at the site of rupture of a nonobstructive lipid rich atherosclerotic plaque that is surrounded by inflammation and a thin fibrous cap. Most of these "vulnerable" plaques are not hemodynamically significant before rupture. A partially occluding (platelet-rich) thrombus that impairs coronary blood flow may lead to *unstable angina.* Therapy with antiplatelet agents (e.g., aspirin, clopidogrel, GP IIB/IIIA receptor inhibitor) is most effective at this time. An intermittently occlusive thrombus may cause myocardial necrosis, producing a *non-ST elevation (non-Q-wave) MI* (non-STEMI). If the thrombus totally occludes the coronary artery for a prolonged period, an *ST elevation (Q-wave) MI* (STEMI) results. The clot is rich in thrombin. Early reperfusion therapy by means of prompt fibrinolysis (along with

Figure 16-2

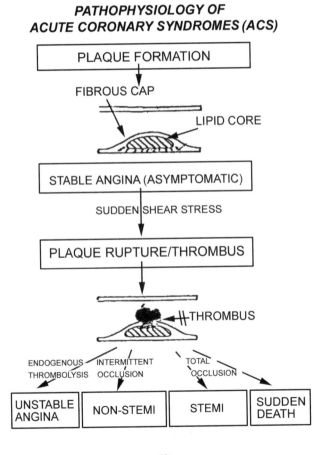

unfractionated or low molecular weight heparin) or direct PCI may limit infarct size and prevent *sudden cardiac death*.

The treatment of patients with CAD should be directed toward both the alleviation of symptoms and an improvement in prognosis. In general, this involves several approaches to modify lifestyle and risk factors (e.g., diet, exercise, hypertension, hypercholesterolemia, cigarette smoking, diabetes), along with pharmacologic therapy and coronary revascularization if needed.

The ABCs of secondary (preventing a recurrent coronary event in patients with known CAD) prevention:

A: **Antiplatelet therapy.** Aspirin indefinitely (or clopidogrel, if aspirin contraindicated) in stable CAD. Dual antiplatelet therapy (DAPT), i.e., aspirin plus a P2Y12 inhibitor (clopidogrel, prasugrel, ticagrelor) in ACS or after PCI (to prevent stent thrombosis).
ACE inhibitor or ARB (especially if post-MI with LV ejection fraction <40%, CHF, hypertension, diabetes mellitus, or proteinuric chronic kidney disease)

B: **Beta blockers** (for up to 3 years post-MI or if LV ejection fraction <40%)
Blood Pressure control (to achieve a goal BP <130/80 mmHg if tolerated)

C: **Cholesterol-lowering therapy** with high intensity "statins" (e.g., atorvastatin 80 mg), if tolerated (to achieve a >50% reduction in LDL cholesterol)
Cardiac rehabilitation (for patients with a recent cardiac event or procedure)
Cigarette smoking cessation (including counseling, nicotine replacement therapy, bupropion, varenicline, and formal cessation program)

D: **Diet.** In general, no more than 25–35% of total calories should come from fat, 15% from protein, and 50–60% from carbohydrates, preferably complex. In addition, less than 7% of the calories should come from saturated fats (including *trans*-fatty acids in products, e.g., margarine and commercial baked goods). The latest dietary recommendations from the American Heart Association emphasize the intake of fruits, vegetables, and whole grains, reduction of sweets and salt (if hypertensive), maintenance of normal body weight, and the intake of monounsaturated and polyunsaturated fats, especially oily fish rich in omega-3 fatty acids, and fiber.
Diabetes management with lifestyle modification and metformin (a biguanide) to achieve a hemoglobin [Hb] A1c <7%. Consider adding empagliflozin (a sodium glucose cotransporter 2 inhibitor) or liraglutide (a glucagon-like peptide-1 agonist) to reduce cardiovascular risk. Avoid thioglitazones if CHF is present.

E: **Exercise and Education.** Exercise can help to lower elevated BP, LDL cholesterol, and triglyceride levels, raise low HDL cholesterol, improve glucose control, and reduce weight (the major abnormalities comprising the *metabolic syndrome*), along with stress, anxiety and depression. When you counsel a patient with heart disease about physical activity, remember to advise him or her to avoid extremes of exertion and extremes of weather (e.g., bitter-cold, hot-humid). Sexual activity, including the potential dangers involved in treating erectile dysfunction with drugs e.g., sildenafil (Viagra) should be discussed openly with a patient (and significant other) who has heart disease. Most patients can resume sexual activity shortly after returning home from an acute MI or after treatment for other cardiac problems, including cardiac surgery.

F: **Flu and Pneumococcal vaccine** (recommended for all patients with cardiovascular disease).

Note: Hormone replacement therapy in older postmenopausal women, antioxidant vitamins C, E, and beta carotene, folic acid with or without vitamins B6 and B12 (aimed at lowering homocysteine), antibiotic treatment (directed against chlamydia pneumoniae), and chelation therapy are not recommended for the secondary prevention of CAD.

ANGINA PECTORIS

Angina pectoris is most commonly caused by the inability of narrowed atherosclerotic coronary arteries to supply oxygen to the heart muscle under conditions of increased myocardial oxygen demand.

Management of Stable Angina Pectoris

The goals of treatment are to provide symptomatic relief of angina and decreased cardiovascular events and mortality, if possible. All patients with angina pectoris should initially be evaluated for a contributing reversible cause. These may include hypertension, CHF, anemia, hypoxemia, sympathomimetic drugs (e.g., vasoconstrictors, inhaled beta agonists, theophylline), and thyrotoxicosis. Medical therapy focuses on increasing coronary blood supply, reducing myocardial oxygen demand, along with stabilization of the atherosclerotic plaque.

Sublingual or oral spray nitroglycerin (for immediate relief) should be prescribed. Patients should be instructed to take one tablet or spray every 5 minutes up to a total of 3 doses, in the sitting or reclining position (to avoid symptomatic postural hypotension), when an anginal attack occurs. Nitroglycerin may also be used prophylactically before an anticipated episode of angina. Although prompt response to nitroglycerin is characteristic of stable angina and is a useful diagnostic consideration in the history, it is important to keep in mind that esophageal spasm and gastroesophageal reflux disease, and even some psychogenic causes of chest pain, may also respond to nitroglycerin. Also, old nitroglycerin can lose its potency over time. Remember to tell your patients to keep the nitroglycerin tablets in the original, dark glass bottle that they came in, and that they should be replaced every 3–6 months. There is much less chance of deterioration of their potency if they are kept in glass, stored in a cool, dry place, and the cotton plug is removed and left out. Avoid fancy or expensive pill containers (occasionally referred to as "gizmos"), often embroidered with jewels, and made of silver or gold. Nitroglycerin tablets are very sensitive and lose their potency when exposed to light, heat, or moisture (Note: nitroglycerin spray may retain potency for up to 3 years.) Keep in mind that if the patient no longer obtains relief of ischemic chest discomfort, and/or doesn't experience the usual "sting", "flushing", "fullness of the head", or "headache", it could be a clue that the medication is too old rather than a sign of unstable angina, which often doesn't respond to NTG, or some other non-coronary condition. A surprising number of patients who have seen a practitioner in the past for typical angina pectoris have never been given a prescription for sublingual or oral spray nitroglycerin! If the pain lasts longer, they should chew an aspirin (if not contraindicated) and be transported immediately to an emergency department for evaluation. Beta blockers (to reduce cardiac oxygen demand) are effective as initial therapy, in the absence of contraindications, to reduce anginal symptoms. Since beta blockers have been shown to reduce reinfarction and prolong life in patients with a prior MI or CHF, these agents are a reasonable first choice. The most commonly used beta blockers are atenolol (Tenormin) and metoprolol (Lopressor, Toprol XL). In patients unable to tolerate beta blockers (e.g., due to severe reactive airway disease), a calcium channel blocker (e.g., diltiazem, verapamil), for coronary vasodilation, is a reasonable alternative therapy. In patients with continued angina, combination therapy should be considered. Such therapy includes a beta blocker and a vasodilating calcium channel blocker (e.g., amlodipine, long-acting nifedipine) or an oral long-acting nitrate preparation (e.g., Imdur, Ismo, Isordil). These agents improve the myocardial oxygen supply/demand balance and therefore reduce symptoms and improve exercise tolerance. The most important factor in using oral (or transdermal) nitrates is to allow for a nitrate-free interval of 8–10 hours to avoid nitrate tolerance.

The type of anginal syndrome the patient has determines the kind of anti-ischemic therapy. For example, *beta blockers* (by decreasing heart rate, BP, and contractility, and thus, myocardial oxygen demand) are more likely to be effective in patients with "*fixed threshold*" angina (where the fixed, narrowed coronary artery results in an angina that increases with increased oxygen demand), whereas *calcium channel blockers and nitrates* (by dilating the coronary arteries) are very effective in preventing the spasms of *variant (Prinzmetal's) angina* (where unexpected spasms of the coronary artery result in ischemia). Beta blockers, on the other hand, by leaving the α receptors that mediate vasoconstriction unopposed, may worsen Prinzmetal's angina and increase the duration of the attacks. A careful clinical history, therefore, may not only indicate the cause of chest pain (i.e., ischemia) but may also provide a clue as to the potential underlying mechanism and advisable treatment.

In addition to controlling the patient's symptoms, consider secondary prevention interventions that stabilize the atherosclerotic plaque and decrease the risk of CAD progression and future cardiac events. These include aspirin (or clopidogrel if aspirin-allergic), a "heart healthy" diet, cholesterol-reduction therapy with high intensity "statins", if tolerated, along with exercise (30-60 minutes 5–7 days per week), smoking cessation, and control of hypertension (BP goal <130/80 mmHg if tolerated) and hyperglycemia (HbA1c <7%).

Patients with symptoms that significantly interfere with their quality of life despite medical treatment, and those with a markedly positive stress test that suggests they are at high risk for future cardiac events, should undergo cardiac catheterization with plans for myocardial revascularization (e.g., PCI, CABG) if anatomically-suitable lesions are found. Survival after the onset of angina pectoris depends on several factors, including the location, severity, and extent of coronary arteries involved by the atherosclerotic process, and the state of LV function. PCI may provide symptomatic relief in some patients with stable angina who are refractory to, or unable to tolerate, medical therapy, but does not decrease the future risk of MI or death (as it does in patients with ACS).

CABG provides excellent relief from symptoms (partial relief in >90% of patients and complete relief in >70%) in patients unresponsive to medical management. CABG also increases survival in those at high risk, i.e., with left main, triple vessel disease or double vessel disease involving the proximal portion of the left anterior descending coronary artery associated with depressed LV function, especially if diabetic.

Occasionally, a patient has severe angina despite medical therapy and/or PCI/CABG. Such a patient may derive symptom improvement with *ranolazine* (Ranexa), a novel antianginal agent that inhibits late sodium entry into ischemic myocardial cells, which reduces calcium overload and LV wall tension, and improves myocardial relaxation and perfusion.

Ongoing medical treatment for stable angina pectoris includes risk factor modification, including statins (which may stabilize plaques and make them less prone to rupture), aspirin, nitrates, beta blockers, and calcium channel blockers. The goal of therapy is to abolish or reduce anginal attacks of myocardial ischemia and to promote a normal life style. *Remember, however, that nitrates and calcium channel blockers can relieve, but beta blockers may worsen, chest pain in patients with variant or Prinzmetal's angina caused by coronary artery spasm (beta blockers prevent vasodilation due to unopposed alpha-vasoconstriction).*

Figure 16-3 summarizes the pharmacologic therapy of stable angina pectoris.

Management of Unstable Angina

Individuals with unstable angina have a greater risk of developing MI or dying suddenly than do patients with stable angina. If untreated, unstable angina progresses to nonfatal MI in 10–20% and death in 5–10% of patients. Most of these events occur within days to weeks after symptom onset. Because unstable angina is a potentially serious development, hospitalization for stabilization, assessment, and more aggressive invasive management strategies than for chronic stable angina is often necessary. Acute treatment includes measures to restore balance between myocardial oxygen supply and demand (e.g., beta blockers, nitrates, and/or calcium channel blockers) and stabilization of the intracoronary thrombus (e.g., aspirin and/or clopidogrel, IV unfractionated or subcutaneous (SQ) low molecular weight heparin).

- All patients with unstable angina should be treated promptly with aspirin and/or clopidogrel, if aspirin is contraindicated due to hypersensitivity or intolerance, as well as an antithrombin agent, e.g., IV unfractionated

Figure 16-3

PHARMACOLOGIC THERAPY OF ANGINA PECTORIS

DRUG CLASS	ANTIANGINAL EFFECT	SIDE EFFECTS
Organic Nitrates (SL, topical, oral)	↓ Myocardial oxygen demand: ↓ Preload > afterload ↑ Oxygen supply: Coronary vasodilation	Headache, hypotension, reflex tachycardia, flushing, tolerance develops with continued use.
β -blockers (e.g., atenolol, metoprolol, nadolol, propranolol)	↓ Myocardial oxygen demand ↓ Heart rate ↓ BP ↓ Contractility	May aggravate bradycardia, heart block, and CHF, provoke bronchospasm, fatigue, depression, cold hands and feet, vivid dreams, and impotence, may worsen dyslipidemia and mask the symptoms of hypoglycemia. Avoid in Prinzmetal's (vasospastic) angina–can provoke coronary artery spasm and aggravate peripheral vascular disease.
Calcium channel blockers Dihydropyridines (e.g., nifedipine, amlodipine) Nondihydropyridines (e.g., verapamil, diltiazem)	↓ Myocardial oxygen demand ↓ Preload ↓ Heart rate (verapamil, diltiazem) ↓ BP ↓ Contractility (verapamil, diltiazem) ↑ Oxygen supply Coronary vasodilation	Headache, flushing, peripheral edema. May worsen CHF, and aggravate bradycardia (verapamil, diltiazem), AV block and hypotension. Constipation (verapamil). Short acting formulations (nifedipine) may provoke reflex tachycardia and aggravate angina.
Late sodium current inhibitor (e.g., ranolazine)	↓ Myocardial oxygen demand ↓ LV diastolic wall tension. No effect on heart rate or BP ↑ Oxygen supply ↓ Compression of the small intramural blood vessels	Prolongs the QT interval. Avoid in patients with long QT interval, on QT prolonging drugs, or with liver disease. Approved for use with nitrates, β-blockers, or amlodipine, limit dose with diltiazem or verapamil (which increases the plasma level of ranolazine).

67

heparin or SQ low molecular weight heparin. A direct thrombin inhibitor, e.g., IV bivalirudin, or a Factor Xa inhibitor, e.g., SQ fondaparinux, may be acceptable alternatives for patients undergoing an invasive or more conservative medical strategy, respectively.

- In higher risk ACS patients (e.g., ST depression, increased troponin levels), a more rapid and potent antiplatelet agent than clopidogrel, e.g., prasugrel (at the time of PCI only) or ticagrelor, and/or GP IIb/IIIa inhibitors (GPIs) should be considered. IV cangrelor may be considered as an adjunct to PCI in patients not receiving oral P2Y12 inhibitors or planned GPIs. When used appropriately, these agents have been shown to reduce adverse events (e.g., death, MI, recurrent ischemia). The GPIs currently approved for use "upstream", with or without PCI, include eptifibatide and tirofiban. Abciximab is reserved for use only with PCI. Optimal timing of therapy has not yet been established. Although a theoretical advantage of starting therapy "upstream" is that it allows patients with recurrent ischemia who are awaiting intervention to benefit from the drug, it may well be appropriate perform diagnostic angiography as expeditiously as possible, and administer therapy in the cath lab (especially if large thrombus burden is present) since no clear benefit of routinely starting GPIs prior to PCI has been demonstrated, and there is an increased risk of bleeding. Contraindications to the use of GP IIb/IIIa inhibitors generally include those factors that predispose patients to increased bleeding risks (e.g., active bleeding, prior intracranial hemorrhage, a history of recent stroke, recent major surgery or trauma, low platelet count).

- Sublingual (tablet or spray), IV and/or oral nitrates should be administered for recurrent episodes of angina. IV and/or oral beta blocker therapy should be considered (if no contraindications exist). When beta-blockers are not tolerated and/or contraindicated, a nondihydropyridine (rate-slowing) calcium channel blocker (e.g., diltiazem or verapamil) may be considered, in the absence of severe LV dysfunction (due to their myocardial depressant effects) or other contraindications. For patients who have recurrent angina despite adequate beta blocker and nitrate therapy, consider a vasodilating calcium channel blocker, e.g., amlodipine (Norvasc).

- *High risk* ACS patients (**Figure 16-4**) should undergo an early invasive strategy (cardiac catheterization within 24 hours with plans for revascularization, if the anatomy is suitable). Patients who are at a *lower risk* and who are clinically stable can be treated more conservatively. They may undergo noninvasive exercise or pharmacologic stress testing (along with nuclear or echo imaging) or coronary CT angiography to screen for provocable ischemia or CAD. In many cases, those patients who have not experienced recurrent chest pain and have no ECG changes, no cardiac enzyme elevations, and/or no evidence of ischemia on exercise testing or imaging procedures, may be discharged directly from the emergency department (ED) (or chest pain observation unit).

Figure 16-4

HIGH-RISK FEATURES OF ACS

- Accelerating tempo of ischemic symptoms (within 48 hours)
- Prolonged ongoing rest pain
- New ST-segment depression (or transient elevation)
- Elevated troponin levels (indicates cardiac necrosis)
- Recurrent angina or ischemia at rest or with low-level activity despite intensive anti-ischemic therapy
- Recurrent angina or ischemia with symptoms of congestive heart failure, an S3 gallop, pulmonary edema, worsening rales, or new or worsening mitral regurgitation
- High-risk findings on noninvasive stress testing
- Ejection fraction < 40%
- Hemodynamic instability (e.g., hypotension, tachycardia)
- Sustained ventricular tachycardia
- Percutaneous coronary intervention within 6 months
- Previous coronary artery bypass graft surgery
- Post-MI angina

- After stabilizing the patient by medication or revascularization, the subsequent long-term treatment should aim at preventing recurrence of episodes of angina and/or MI, and at halting the progression of CAD. An ACE inhibitor should be considered when hypertension, LV systolic dysfunction, or diabetes mellitus is present, along with lipid lowering therapy with high intensity "statins", if tolerated. Specific instructions should be given to the patient regarding smoking cessation, diet, exercise, achievement of optimal weight, hypertension control (to a BP goal of <130/80 mmHg, if tolerated), and control of hyperglycemia if diabetic (HbA1c <7%).

Since in unstable angina, the vessel usually remains patent and the thrombi are undergoing continuous spontaneous formation and thrombolysis, *thrombolytic therapy has not been shown to be effective in improving the outcome* and is not recommended.

"To medicate, to dilate, or to operate?"—That is the question: Opinions vary concerning the indications for pharmacologic, interventional, and/or surgical solutions to CAD. However, most would agree that the following patients should be considered for CABG: those with debilitating angina pectoris on medical therapy; those with significant left main, triple vessel, and double vessel CAD involving the proximal portion of the left anterior descending coronary artery, accompanied by decreased LV function (especially if diabetic); and those with ongoing unstable angina or ischemia and/or hemodynamic instability following a failed PCI. Whenever possible, arterial conduits (e.g., internal mammary, radial) should be utilized since their long-term patency rate is far better than for saphenous vein grafts. The

availability of drug-eluting stents (DES) (which greatly reduce restenosis) has shifted the paradigm to more PCIs. Concerns over the risk of late stent thrombosis (which is less with newer generation DES) and data demonstrating that PCI, with newer generation DES, in addition to relieving symptoms, offers an advantage over older generation DES and bare metal stents (BMS) in reducing the risk of stent thrombosis, restenosis, and repeat target vessel revascularization, has added fuel to the debate.

Figure 16-5 summarizes the treatment of ACS. The main aims of treatment are to alleviate symptoms, prolong life, reduce myocardial damage, and prevent recurrences.

Figure 16-5

THERAPY IN ACUTE CORONARY SYNDROMES (ACS)

I. ANTIPLATELET AGENTS

Aspirin (chewed, swallowed) – a cyclooxygenase (COX) inhibitor
—Reduces mortality alone or in conjunction with thrombolysis (for ST segment elevation MI)
—Reduces recurrent ischemia, reocclusion, and reinfarction.

Clopidogrel (Plavix) – an irreversible thienopyridine ADP (P2Y12) receptor antagonist
—If aspirin contraindicated (e.g., intolerance, allergy)
—Reduces mortality and MI in combination with aspirin in non-ST elevation MI, and improves infarct-related artery patency and reduces ischemic complications when combined with aspirin and fibrinolytic therapy in ST elevation MI
—Prevents thrombotic complications following PCI (stenting). Recent data suggests decreased antiplatelet effect when clopidogrel is combined with proton pump inhibitors, particularly omeprazole and esomeprazole.

Prasugrel (Effient) – an irreversible thienopyridine ADP (P2Y12) receptor antagonist
—More rapid, potent, and consistent platelet inhibition than clopidogrel.
—Fewer atherothrombotic events when compared with clopidogrel in high risk ACS patients undergoing PCI, albeit at an increased risk of significant bleeding. Use with caution in patients > 75 years of age and those with low body weight (< 60 kg). Contraindicated in patients with history of prior TIA or stroke.

Ticagrelor (Brilinta) – a reversible cyclopentyltriazolopyrimidine ADP (P2Y12) receptor antagonist
—More potent and consistent platelet inhibition than clopidogrel with more rapid "onset" and "offset" of action
—Fewer vascular deaths, MIs, and stent thromboses than clopidogrel in ACS patients with or without ST elevation, without an increase in overall major bleeding, but with an increase in non-CABG related bleeding. Unique side effects include dyspnea and ventricular pauses (thought to be adenosine

mediated). Maintenance dose of aspirin above 100 mg daily may decrease the effectiveness of ticagrelor and should be avoided.

Glycoprotein IIb/IIIa receptor antagonist – e.g., abciximab (ReoPro), eptifibatide (Integrilin), tirofiban (Aggrastat)

—Reduces mortality, MI, and recurrent ischemia in high risk ACS patients, especially those undergoing PCI. Eptifibatide and tirofiban are approved for use with or without PCI, whereas abciximab is indicated only with PCI. Abciximab remains the agent of choice in patients at highest risk (e.g., diabetes, renal insufficiency, ST elevation MI), especially those with large clot burden at the time of PCI. Thrombocytopenia can occur, and may require discontinuation of the drug +/– platelet transfusion.

—Use of these agents in combination with reduced dose fibrinolytic therapy in acute ST elevation MI does not confer a mortality benefit, and is associated with an increased risk of bleeding. Decreased dose adjustments for eptifibatide and tirofiban (not abciximab) are required in patients with reduced renal function.

II. ANTICOAGULANTS

Heparin (unfractionated)—IV bolus and drip

—Maintains vessel patency and reduces reocclusion, particularly in conjunction with fibrin-specific thrombolytic agents (e.g., tPA, reteplase, tenecteplase (probably not necessary after streptokinase) and for all patients undergoing direct or adjunctive PCI.

—Reduces mortality and MI (in pre-fibrinolytic era)

—Requires monitoring of PTT levels.

—Sensitivity to heparin may be decreased when it is used concomitantly with IV nitroglycerin (higher doses may be needed to achieve anticoagulation effect).

Low Molecular Weight Heparin–SQ – e.g., enoxaparin (Lovenox), dalteparin (Fragmin).

—Does not usually require laboratory monitoring of activity.

—Enoxaparin approved for prevention of ischemic complications in unstable angina and non ST segment elevation MI when used with aspirin (can be "advantageously" substituted for IV unfractionated heparin (UFH) in the absence of renal failure, unless CABG is planned within 24 hours). Recent evidence favors use of enoxaparin with full dose TNK-tPA in ST elevation MI (in patients < 75 years of age without significant renal dysfunction). Enoxaparin may be a reasonable alternative to UFH for PCI anticoagulation, but has not been shown to be superior to UFH during PCI for preventing ischemic complications.

Direct Thrombin Inhibitors, e.g., IV bivalirudin (Angiomax) and **Factor Xa Inhibitors**, e.g., SQ fondaparinux (Arixtra), a synthetic heparin analog, may be acceptable alternatives to UFH or enoxaparin in patients with ACS. Bivalirudin is also approved for use in patients with, or at risk of, HIT undergoing PCI. Before PCI, UFH must be added to fondaparinux to lessen risk of catheter thrombosis. Fondaparinux does not require laboratory monitoring of its anticoagulant effect. Thrombocytopenia can occur, but HIT has not yet been reported.

Figure 16-5

THERAPY IN ACUTE CORONARY SYNDROMES (ACS) (*Continued*)

Warfarin (Coumadin)
—Prevents thromboembolism, particularly useful in larger anterior MI, with LV mural thrombus, congestive heart failure, apical dyskinesis or aneurysm formation, and atrial fibrillation.
—Evidence suggests warfarin reduces reinfarction and late mortality.

III. ANTI-ISCHEMIC THERAPY

Nitroglycerin (IV, oral)
—acute phase: No effect on survival. (The value of routine administration of IV nitroglycerin to patients also receiving fibrinolytic therapy is indeterminate).
—reduces myocardial oxygen demand: dilates systemic arteries (reduces afterload) and veins (reduces preload).
—increases myocardial oxygen supply: dilates infarct-related coronary vessels, improves collateral blood flow, relieves coronary spasm (spontaneous or cocaine-induced).
—useful for ischemic chest pain, hypertension, CHF, attenuation of LV expansion and remodeling (large anterior MI).
—may be hazardous if hypotension (BP < 90 mmHg) develops, especially in inferior MI complicated by RV infarction (reduced coronary perfusion pressure → worsens myocardial ischemia).
—tolerance may develop after 24 hours of continuous IV therapy.
—avoid use of nitroglycerin in patients who have taken sildenafil (Viagra), vardenafil (Levitra), or tadalafil (Cialis) within 24–48 hours (refractory hypotension and death have been reported).

Beta-blockers (IV, oral)
—acute phase: proven mortality benefit with or without thrombolysis.
—decreases myocardial oxygen demand (↓ HR, ↓ BP, ↓ contractility).
—decreases infarct size, recurrent ischemia, reinfarction, incidence of cardiac rupture, ventricular tachycardia and fibrillation, and mortality.
—useful if hyperdynamic state (tachycardia, hypertension) and ongoing chest pain.
—contraindications include severe hypotension, bradycardia, decompensated LV failure, reactive airway disease, recent cocaine use (controversial).

Calcium Channel Blockers
—acute phase: no proven mortality benefit (or actual harm) for all calcium channel blockers.
—limited role post-MI
—diltiazem: may be beneficial in preventing reinfarction and recurrent angina in subset of patients with non-Q wave MI and intact LV function–

72

detrimental effect noted, however, in subset of patients with LV dysfunction (pulmonary congestion or ejection fraction <40%).

—verapamil: use in late phase (2nd week after acute MI) shown to reduce reinfarction and mortality in patients without heart failure—neither benefit observed, however, in patients with heart failure.

—calcium channel blockers may be considered for post-infarction angina and hypertension (after the acute phase) in beta blocker intolerant patient without congestive heart failure and/or LV dysfunction (since they reduce ventricular contractility), and for ACS precipitated by cocaine use.

IV. OTHER

Angiotensin Converting Enzyme (ACE) Inhibitors or Angiotensin Receptor Blockers (ARBs)

—acute phase: confers mortality benefit particularly in high-risk groups (e.g., large anterior MI).

—attenuates LV dilation, myocardial remodeling, and aneurysm formation.

—reduces incidence of CHF and recurrent MI in patients with ejection fraction ≤ 40%.

HMG CoA reductase Inhibitors ("statins")

—High intensity statins, e.g., atorvastatin (Lipitor) 40-80 mg and rosuvastatin (Crestor) 20-40 mg should be administered to reduce LDL cholesterol by at least 50%, if tolerated. Statins have also been shown to be beneficial in reducing vascular inflammation, improving endothelial dysfunction, stabilizing impending plaque rupture, and reducing CAD events and mortality (so-called "pleiotropic effects").

Nonstatin lipid lowering agents, e.g., ezetimibe (Zetia) and PCSK9 inhibitors, e.g., alirocumab (Praluent) and evolocumab (Repatha), have been shown to further reduce cardiovascular event rates, and may be added to maximally tolerated statin therapy if LDL cholesterol remains ≥ 70 mg/dL ("lower is better").

Cardiac catheterization and coronary intervention

—Reduces recurrent ischemia, MI, and mortality when compared with medical therapy alone, especially in high risk ACS patients.

—includes angioplasty/stenting (for patients with anatomically suitable stenoses), or bypass surgery for patients with significant left main, triple-vessel or double-vessel disease (involving the proximal portion of the left anterior descending artery [LAD]) with depressed LV function, especially if diabetic.

ACUTE MYOCARDIAL INFARCTION

Acute myocardial infarction (MI) is a common, often dramatic and potentially fatal form of ACS characterized by a rise and/or fall in cardiac biomarkers (preferably troponin) together with clinical, ECG, and/or imaging evidence suggestive of ischemic myocardial necrosis. MIs may be classified into five types based on whether they are: 1) caused by a primary coronary event (i.e., ACS), 2) secondary to a supply-demand ischemic imbalance, with or without underlying CAD, 3) resulting in sudden cardiac death, 4) related to a PCI procedure, or 5) associated with CABG surgery. Acute MI related to ACS (so-called "type 1" MI) typically results from rupture of a "vulnerable" atherosclerotic plaque (characterized by a lipid-rich core, surrounding inflammation, and a thin overlying fibrous cap) with superimposed occlusive (ST elevation MI) or non-occlusive (non-ST elevation MI) intracoronary thrombus formation. Slowly developing high-grade coronary artery stenoses usually do not precipitate acute MI because of the development of adequate collateral circulation over time. Instead, plaques prone to rupture often are only mild to moderately stenotic (i.e., not flow limiting) and, therefore, generally do not cause clinical angina. Of note, acute MI can also occur secondary to a supply-demand ischemic mismatch (so-called "type-2" MI), e.g., from anemia, tachyarrhythmias, hypo- or hypertension. Since the extent of myocardial necrosis (with its resultant heart failure, myocardial rupture, and associated ventricular tachyarrhythmias) plays a crucial role in the prognosis and can be successfully treated if diagnosed early, it is essential that the clinician rapidly and accurately establish the diagnosis of acute MI. Then, acute interventions, i.e., PCI/thrombolysis (for "type 1" MI) or therapy directed at the underlying cause (for "type 2" MI) may be initiated to suitable patients as soon as possible.

An accurate and focused clinical history should be obtained as quickly as possible, including investigation as to the indications and potential contraindications to thrombolytic therapy (**Figure 16-7**).

Management of Acute MI

In patients who present with an ST elevation MI, the importance of immediate patient evaluation and prompt initiation of reperfusion therapies (i.e., thrombolytic agents, PCI) cannot be over-emphasized. Overall, mortality is decreased ~ 25–30% when reperfusion therapy is given early. The sooner the reperfusion is administered, the better. If treatment is initiated within the first 3 hours, a 50% or greater reduction in mortality can be achieved. The greater the amount of time that lapses from the onset of chest pain to reperfusion, the greater the loss of viable, functional myocardium which, in turn, results in an increase in morbidity and mortality. Although the magnitude of benefit declines rapidly over time, a 10% relative mortality reduction can still be achieved up to 12 hours after the onset of chest pain. The ultimate goal in patients with acute ST segment elevation MI (or new LBBB) who are within 6 to 12 hours of the onset of symptoms is initiation of

Figure 16-7

THROMBOLYTIC THERAPY FOR ACUTE ST SEGMENT ELEVATION MI

Patient Selection

A. Indications

- Clinical history of chest pain (or its equivalent) compatible with acute MI and unresponsive to nitroglycerin.
- ST segment elevation ≥1 mm in 2 or more contiguous ECG leads, or new (or presumably new) left bundle branch block (LBBB).*
- <6 hours after symptoms onset (<3 hours most beneficial).
- 6–12 hours (still beneficial), especially if ongoing ischemic chest pain, high-risk patient with large amount of myocardium in jeopardy (extensive anterior MI, inferior MI with precordial ST depression and/or RV infarction).
- Controversial: 12–24 hours after pain onset. Non-ST segment elevation MI does not appear to benefit; however, anterior ST depression MI with prominent R wave in leads V2–V3 (left circumflex or true posterior MI) may benefit.

B. Major Contraindications

- Active or recent (within 2–4 weeks) internal bleeding (excluding menses)
- Suspected aortic dissection, or acute pericarditis.
- Recent(<6 weeks) surgical procedure; head trauma; prolonged (>10 minutes) or traumatic CPR.
- History of cerebrovascular accident–hemorrhagic stroke (ever), thrombotic stroke (<12 months), seizures or intracranial mass, neoplasm, AV malformation or aneurysm.
- Known bleeding diathesis or current use of anticoagulants (INR > 2–3).
- Severe uncontrolled hypertension (systolic BP >180, diastolic BP >110 mmHg).
- Previous allergic reaction to the chosen thrombolytic agent, e.g., streptokinase (SK)—infrequently used in current practice.

Note: Time is muscle! All available thrombolytic agents restore coronary blood flow, limit infarct size, preserve LV function and reduce attendant morbidity and mortality. The choice of agent is much less important to survival than is the wider use of reperfusion therapy (PCI/thrombolysis) and the delay time to initiation of treatment. When thrombolytic therapy is chosen as the primary reperfusion strategy, it should be administered within 30 minutes of hospital arrival ("door-to-needle" time). Direct PCI is the preferred reperfusion strategy when available within 90 minutes of presentation ("door-to-balloon" time), or within 120 minutes if transfer to a PCI-capable hospital is required.

*In patients who present with chest pain and a presumed new anterior STEMI, ST elevation in V2-V3 ≥ 2 mm in men or ≥ 1.5 mm in women improves the diagnostic accuracy. In patients with LBBB, highly specific, but poorly sensitive, ECG criteria can be used to more accurately diagnose a STEMI: (1) ST elevation ≥1 mm and *concordant* (in the same direction) with the QRS (strongest predictor); (2) ST depression ≥1 mm and *concordant* in leads V1, V2, or V3; and (3) ST elevation ≥ 5 mm and *excessively discordant* (in the opposite direction) with the QRS (weakest predictor) – "Sgarbossa's criteria."

fibrinolytic therapy within 30 minutes of hospital arrival ("door-to-needle" time), or even sooner during transport, or direct PCI within 90 minutes of first medical contact ("door to balloon time"), or 120 minutes if transfer to a PCI-capable hospital is required. Direct PCI should be considered the preferred approach, particularly when the patient presents >3 hours after symptom onset, in cardiogenic shock or severe heart failure, or when thrombolytic therapy is contraindicated or the diagnosis is in doubt. Although direct PCI may be preferable, only a minority of hospitals in the U.S. have this capability on an emergency basis, and as a result, thrombolytic therapy is the most commonly used method (when indicated) for attempting reperfusion of a totally occluded infarct-related artery (**Figure 16-8**).

At present, a conservative management strategy (including noninvasive evaluation of LV function and a modified exercise stress test with or without nuclear or echo imaging) is being used for most patients after successful thrombolysis for ST elevation MI, and for many patients with non ST elevation MI. After thrombolytic therapy has been administered, emergency PCI is currently reserved for high risk patients with ongoing pain, spontaneous or inducible ischemia, significantly reduced LV function (with "viable" myocardium), or electrical and/or hemodynamic instability. Of note, recent data has demonstrated a beneficial effect of routine early PCI after successful fibrinolysis for patients with ST elevation MI.

All patients with chest pain and/or symptoms compatible with acute MI ≤ 12 hours in duration, with ST elevation or new (or presumably new) LBBB, should promptly receive 162-325 mg non-enteric coated aspirin (chewed initially to quicken absorption), and/or clopidogrel (if aspirin contraindicated), ticagrelor, or prasugrel (if PCI planned). They should also receive an anti-thrombin agent, e.g., IV unfractionated heparin or SQ LMWH (enoxaparin [Lovenox]) to prevent rethrombosis, particularly if a clot-specific agent (e.g., accelerated alteplase [tPA], reteplase [rPA], tenecteplase [TNK-tPA]) is used for thrombolytic therapy. Patients at high risk for systemic emboli (e.g., large anterior MI, atrial fibrillation, LV thrombus) are also candidates for antithrombin therapy. Primary PCI, in conjunction with IV unfractionated heparin (with or without GP IIb/IIIa inhibitors [GPIs]), or bivalirudin (if bleeding risk is high), and the selective (no benefit of routine) use of manual aspiration thrombectomy (if large thrombus burden), is the preferred reperfusion strategy in patients with acute ST elevation MI, as it is associated with lower rates of reinfarction, mortality, and intracranial bleeding when compared to thrombolytic therapy.

After primary PCI, low dose aspirin is continued indefinitely, along with a prolonged course of P2Y12 inhibitor (ticagrelor or prasugrel preferred over clopidogrel) to reduce the risk of ischemic complications and stent thrombosis.

Routine use of a GPI is not recommended in patients who have received fibrinolytics or in those receiving bivalirudin because of an increased risk of bleeding.

ACC/AHA guidelines recommend that SQ LMWH (enoxaparin [Lovenox]) can be "advantageously" substituted for IV unfractionated heparin (UFH) in patients with unstable angina and non-ST segment elevation MI, unless CABG is planned within 24 hours, in which case UFH is preferred (since it has a shorter half life than LMWH and can be rapidly reversed with protamine).

Figure 16-8

COMPARISON OF THROMBOLYSIS AND DIRECT PERCUTANEOUS CORONARY INTERVENTION FOR ST SEGMENT ELEVATION MYOCARDIAL INFARCTION

THROMBOLYSIS	PERCUTANEOUS CORONARY INTERVENTION
Universally available	Available only in specialized centers with 24 hr cath lab capability and skilled interventional personnel
Easy, rapid administration	Technologically demanding, time delay to perform. Single-stage procedure. Clot and plaque addressed at same time.
Higher bleeding and stroke risk	Lower bleeding and stroke risk
Higher rates of reocclusion and recurrent ischemia	Lower rates of early reocclusion and ischemia
Many contraindications	Few contraindications. Allows reperfusion when thrombolytics are contraindicated
Lower vessel patency rates (TIMI-3 flow rates 55%–60%)*	Higher vessel patency rates (TIMI-3 flow rates >90%)*
Longer length of hospital stay	Shorter length of hospital stay. Improved survival in high risk patients. Greater efficacy for cardiogenic shock. Provides additional information regarding coronary artery anatomy and left ventricular function. Allows risk stratification.**

*Note: Angiographic assessment of coronary blood flow can be semiquantitated using the grading method of the Thrombolysis in Acute MI (TIMI) investigators. TIMI-0 = no flow past obstruction, TIMI-1 = incomplete filling of vessel, TIMI-2 = slow but complete filling of vessel, TIMI-3 = brisk filling of vessel.

**After administration of thrombolytic therapy, all patients, especially those at high risk (extensive ST segment elevation, previous MI, new onset LBBB, tachycardia, or hypotension), should be transferred to a PCI-capable hospital as soon as possible so that PCI can be performed as needed.

When timely PCI is unavailable, the newer fibrinolytics (e.g., double bolus reteplase [rPA], single bolus tenecteplase [TNK-TPA]) are currently favored over the "gold standard" tPA (and the older non-clot selective agent streptokinase) by some experts because of the ease of bolus administration vs. infusion. More recent evidence suggests a therapeutic paradigm shift towards a regimen that combines LMWH (enoxaparin) with full dose tenecteplase. Thrombolytic agents, however, have not been proven effective for non ST segment elevation MI or unstable angina. In fact, there is evidence that these agents may be harmful, and therefore should not be administered in those conditions. Contraindications to thrombolytic therapy include a history of intracranial hemorrhage; active internal bleeding (excluding menses); severe uncontrolled hypertension (BP ≥180/110 mmHg); recent stroke, major surgery or trauma; brain neoplasm, aneurysm or AV malformation; unclear mental status; suspected aortic dissection; and acute pericarditis. When using thrombolytic therapy, adjunctive pharmacologic treatment includes aspirin and/or clopidogrel, beta blockers (in the absence of contraindications), heparin (especially if a fibrin-specific thrombolytic agent [e.g., TPA, rPA, TNK-TPA] is administered), IV nitroglycerin, and ACE inhibitors/ARBs (particularly in patients with diminished LV function [ejection fraction < 40%]).

Irrespective of whether the patient receives thrombolytic therapy or primary PCI, or neither, beta blockers (due to their antiischemic as well as antiarrhythmic influence) should be administered, when hemodynamically stable, unless contraindicated. IV nitroglycerin should be administered to patients with large anterior MI, CHF, hypertension, and/or persistent or recurrent ischemic chest pain. It should be avoided, however, in patients with hypotension and/or RV infarction (where decreasing preload may decrease cardiac output and lead to more hypotension). IV morphine sulfate should be administered if pain is not relieved with nitroglycerin. (Keep in mind the *memory aid:* **"MONA"**— Morphine, Oxygen [if O$_2$ sat < 90%], Nitroglycerin, Aspirin.)

Definitive treatment is to open the infarct-related artery as soon as possible. For patients with acute MI, the greater the amount of time that lapses from the onset of chest pain to initiation of reperfusion therapies, the greater the loss of viable functional heart muscle. Thrombolysis produces the greatest benefit when given within 3 hours of the onset of symptoms, although the patient may still benefit if the drug is given within 12 hours. Since "time is muscle", patients who are eligible should expeditiously receive either thrombolytic therapy ("door-to-needle" time ≤ 30 minutes) or be taken directly to the cath lab for primary PCI, which has been demonstrated to be superior to thrombolytic therapy in expert hands when performed early without prolonged delay (i.e., "door-to-balloon" time ≤ 90 minutes, or ≤ 120 minutes if transfer to a PCI-capable hospital is required). Direct PCI is to be considered when thrombolytic therapy is absolutely contraindicated. "Facilitated" PCI (upstream thrombolysis "on the way to" immediate PCI) offers no advantage over direct PCI, and increases the risk of bleeding, and therefore, is not recommended. "Rescue" PCI is associated with improved outcomes and may be considered after failed thrombolysis. Routine early PCI (within 3-24 hrs) has recently been shown to improve outcomes in ST elevation MI patients following successful fibrinolysis. Noninfarct artery PCI may be considered at the time of primary culprit PCI, or as a staged procedure, in select patients with ST elevation MI and multivessel CAD.

Patients treated after 12 hours should receive appropriate medical therapy, e.g., nitrates, beta blockers, ACE inhibitors (particularly if large anterior MI with decreased LV function and if patient is diabetic [slows progression of nephropathy]). Patients may be considered candidates for reperfusion therapy on an individual basis. ACE inhibitors have been shown to attenuate LV remodeling (i.e., reduce LV dysfunction and dilatation) and slow the progression of CHF and decrease mortality. Oral anticoagulation with warfarin (preferred) or NOAC is recommended if a large anterior MI with extensive dyskinesis and/or LV thrombus (on echo), or atrial fibrillation is present. Prophylactic lidocaine (or other antiarrhythmic agent) and calcium channel blockers have failed to demonstrate benefit and in fact may even be harmful, and therefore should be avoided (see below).

Calcium channel blockers (particularly the dihydropyridines, e.g., nifedipine) have not been shown to be beneficial in the early treatment or secondary prevention of acute MI. These agents may promote reflex tachycardia and hypotension and thereby exacerbate ischemia, and are not considered part of the routine management of MI patients. (Exception: The rate-slowing non-dihydropyridine calcium channel blocker diltiazem has been shown to reduce recurrent MI in patients with a first non-ST elevation (non-Q wave) MI who have intact LV function). Nifedipine and other short-acting formulations may increase morbidity and mortality. Diltiazem and verapamil should be used with caution, if at all, in patients with LV dysfunction, because they reduce ventricular contractility.

The role of routine magnesium sulfate in patients with acute MI is uncertain. It should be given to the patient with hypomagnesemia, especially if polymorphic VT associated with QT prolongation ("torsades de pointes") is present (since hypomagnesemia prolongs the QT interval and predisposes to torsade de pointes).

Complications of acute MI should be managed appropriately and expeditiously. For example:

- Patients with *CHF* should be treated with ACE inhibitors/ARBs, beta blockers (as tolerated), diuretics, and aldosterone antagonists.

- Symptomatic *ventricular arrhythmias* should be treated with beta blockers (lidocaine is no longer recommended prophylactically due to potentially detrimental effects). If refractory, they should be treated with the antiarrhythmic agent amiodarone, procainamide, or lidocaine, and/ or ICD implantation (in patients at high risk of sudden cardiac death).

- *Supraventricular arrhythmias* should be treated with beta blockers (e.g., IV esmolol), diltiazem, verapamil, digoxin.

- *Cardiogenic shock* is the most common cause of death in hospitalized patients with acute MI. Prompt restoration of coronary blood flow (preferably by PCI) can increase survival. IABP can be used in the interim for hemodynamic stabilization.

- *Surgery* or *percutaneous* intervention may be indicated, particularly for acute MR and VSD.

- Nitroglycerin should be used cautiously, if at all, in patients with *inferior MI* who have concomitant *RV infarction*, since profound hypotension may result. Furthermore, nitroglycerin (or nitrates) should not be administered to patients with chest pain who have taken drugs for erectile dysfunction, e.g., *sildenafil* (Viagra), *vardenafil* (Levitra), or *tadalafil* (Cialis) within the previous 24-48 hours. A marked drop in BP and even death may occur. Viagra is also potentially hazardous in patients with CHF and borderline low BP, including patients on multiple antihypertensive drug therapy.

Note: Consider the use of cocaine in a young person who presents with chest pain, particularly following a party. Cocaine may induce coronary spasm, leading to acute MI. The management of *cocaine-induced* MI differs from that of classic MI. Beta blockers, e.g., metoprolol, should be avoided acutely, as these agents may lead to unopposed α-mediated vasoconstriction and worsen myocardial ischemia. Labetalol and carvedilol, however, have combined (alpha)-and (beta)-blocking properties, and can be considered. Benzodiazepines can be used as an anxiolytic to reduce tachycardia and hypertension, along with antiplatelet and antithrombotic therapy, nitrates, calcium channel blockers, and phentolamine (an α-blocker) to relieve coronary spasm. Immediate angiography with PCI (if appropriate) should be considered if chest pain and ST segment elevation persists. PCI is the preferred reperfusion strategy in these patients, as there are usually comorbid features (e.g., seizures, dissection, severe hypertension) that preclude the use of thrombolytic therapy.

ELECTRICAL COMPLICATIONS OF ACUTE MI

Cardiac arrhythmias and conduction disturbances are the most common complications of acute MI (**Figure 16-9**). With initiation of early reperfusion therapy, both brady and tachyarrhythmias will often develop after restored patency of the infarct-related coronary artery (so-called "reperfusion arrhythmias"). The most common rhythm disorder seen after reperfusion with thrombolytic therapy or PCI is an accelerated idioventricular rhythm, so-called "slow VT", occurring at a rate of 60–100 beats/min, which is well tolerated hemodynamically in most patients. It is transient, and usually does not require specific treatment.

Ventricular Arrhythmias

Ventricular arrhythmias (i.e., PVCs, VT or VF) are the most frequently observed rhythm disturbances in acute MI. They reflect the electrical instability of the damaged ischemic myocardium and occur in >90% of patients during the first 72 hours. Electrolyte imbalance (e.g., hypokalemia, hypomagnesemia),

Figure 16-9

MANAGEMENT OF ELECTRICAL COMPLICATIONS OF ACUTE MYOCARDIAL INFARCTION

I. VENTRICULAR TACHYCARDIA/FIBRILLATION

A. Acute Phase (First 48 Hours)

- If hemodynamically unstable electrical cardioversion/defibrillation/cardiopulmonary resuscitation.
- If hemodynamically stable – IV amiodarone (preferred), procainamide, or lidocaine may be used. Lidocaine reduces primary ventricular fibrillation; however routine prophylaxis no longer recommended for all patients since toxicities (increased fatal asystolic events) tend to offset antifibrillatory benefit.
- Beta blockers—reduce incidence of ventricular tachycardia and fibrillation.
- Correct electrolyte imbalance ($\downarrow K^+$, $\downarrow Mg^{++}$), acid-base disturbances, hypoxemia, adverse drug effects.

B. Convalescent Phase (After 48 Hours)

- Beta blockers and amiodarone
- Consider non-drug methods (e.g., wearable defibrillator or ICD, ventricular aneurysm resection, ablation of arrhythmogenic foci, antitachycardia pacemakers, with or without CABG).

II. SUPRAVENTRICULAR TACHYARRHYTHMIAS

- Beta blockers (esmolol), adenosine, verapamil, diltiazem, digoxin—slows ventricular rate.
- Class IA antiarrhythmics (e.g., procainamide) or class III (e.g., sotalol, amiodarone) or
- Synchronized DC electrical cardioversion, if clinically or hemodynamically unstable—restores sinus rhythm.

III. BRADYARRHYTHMIAS AND CONDUCTION DISTURBANCES

- Atropine
  —If symptomatic or hemodynamically unstable (excessive increase in heart rate may worsen ischemia, extend infarction, or promote ventricular tachycardia/ventricular fibrillation).
- Temporary external transcutaneous or transvenous pacemaker.
  —Mobitz Type II 2nd degree AV block
  —Complete heart block
  —New bifascicular block including alternating right and left bundle branch block (LBBB), new RBBB with left anterior or posterior hemiblock, new LBBB with first degree AV block in anterior MI.

81

hypoxemia, adverse drug effects, and increased sympathoadrenal discharge may also play a role.

PVCs and nonsustained (<30 seconds) VT not associated with hemodynamic compromise, are not indicative of increased risk of sudden cardiac death and do not require specific therapy in the acute phase of MI.

Early-onset or "primary" sustained VT is common in the first hours and days after MI, and does not appear to be associated with an increased risk for subsequent mortality if the arrhythmia is rapidly terminated. Late-onset or "secondary" sustained VT occurring after 24–48 hours, however, is associated with a marked increase in mortality. These late-onset ventricular arrhythmias reflect a transmural infarct of substantial size with advanced LV dysfunction and portend a far more ominous prognosis.

Patients with VF (which may occur without any warning arrhythmias) or sustained VT associated with symptoms or hemodynamic compromise should undergo defibrillation or electrical cardioversion immediately. Underlying ischemia and electrolyte abnormalities ($\downarrow$ K$^+$, $\downarrow$ Mg^{++}) should be addressed and corrected. IV amiodarone remains an effective agent for the treatment of symptomatic VT or VF. *Although it reduces primary VF, lidocaine is no longer used as a prophylactic measure*, since the overall incidence of primary VF (in this era of reperfusion therapy and beta blockade) appears to be decreasing, and recent studies have demonstrated a disturbing trend toward an increased number of fatal bradycardic and asystolic cardiac arrests in lidocaine-treated patients. Persistent ventricular arrhythmias (despite the use of IV amiodarone therapy), however, may necessitate the administration of another antiarrhythmic agent, e.g., IV procainamide or lidocaine and/or a more aggressive invasive (i.e., cardiac catheterization, EPS) management strategy (for those who may benefit from revascularization and/or implantation of an ICD).

Supraventricular Arrhythmias

Supraventricular arrhythmias (i.e., PACs, paroxysmal SVT, atrial fibrillation and/ or flutter) may be manifestations of the left atrial distension and pressure rise resulting from LV failure, and as such are associated with an increased infarct size and mortality. These arrhythmias may also occur with pericarditis, excessive sympathetic stimulation, electrolyte disturbances, hypoxia, or atrial infarction. Sinus tachycardia is the most common supraventricular arrhythmia. If it occurs secondary to another cause (e.g., anemia, fever, CHF), the primary problem should be treated first. However, if it appears to be due to sympathetic overstimulation (e.g., fever, pain, anxiety), then treatment with a beta blocker is indicated. PACs occur in 15–30% of patients and usually do not require specific therapy. They are often harbingers of more severe grades of atrial tachyarrhythmias. Atrial fibrillation occurs in up to 15% of patients early after MI, with atrial flutter and paroxysmal SVT occurring much less frequently.

Management of supraventricular arrhythmias in the setting of acute MI is similar to the management in other settings; however the threshold for cardioversion should be lower and the urgency with which the rapid ventricular response is controlled should be greater. When the ventricular response is rapid, an increase in myocardial oxygen demand and decrease in diastolic filling time may produce hemodynamic instability and exacerbate ischemia. Atrial fibrillation or flutter associated with a rapid ventricular response, therefore, should be treated promptly with electrical cardioversion. Pharmacologic agents, e.g., beta blockers, calcium channel blockers, and digoxin, increase the AV block and slow the ventricular rate. Beta blockers are generally the first line agents in acute MI, to control the rapid ventricular response. Diltiazem and verapamil are appropriate alternatives in patients without CHF or significant LV systolic dysfunction, and digoxin for patients with concomitant LV dysfunction. If spontaneous conversion to normal sinus rhythm does not occur, IV unfractionated or SQ low molecular weight heparin therapy (in patients not already receiving it) along with Class IA antiarrhythmic agents (e.g., procainamide) or Class III agents (e.g., amiodarone) (**Figure 11-1**) should be considered. Of the antiarrhythmic agents available, amiodarone is probably the safest in the peri-infarct setting.

Bradyarrhythmias and Conduction Disturbances

Bradyarrhythmias and conduction disturbances are common during the course of acute MI. They are encountered 2–3 times more frequently in inferior than in anterior MIs, and may be due to increased vagal tone or ischemia and/or infarction of conduction tissue. Prognosis and treatment vary greatly, depending on the size and location of infarct, the ventricular response, the degree of AV block, and the patient's clinical status. The most common bradyarrhythmia associated with acute MI is sinus bradycardia which is seen in 20–25% of patients. It is particularly common early in the course of acute inferior MI, or after reperfusion of the right coronary artery. In most patients with acute MI, sinus bradycardia is asymptomatic and requires no treatment. If the heart rate is extremely low (<40 beats/min) or if systemic hypotension is present, IV atropine should be considered. Atropine should be used sparingly and appropriately, however, because of the protective effect of vagal stimulation against VF in the setting of acute MI.

MECHANICAL COMPLICATIONS OF ACUTE MI

Prompt recognition and attention to serious life-threatening arrhythmias and conduction disturbances that complicate acute MI by modern cardiac care units, along with early restoration of coronary artery patency by aggressive reperfusion strategies, have significantly reduced the in-hospital mortality to 5–10%. The current mortality is almost entirely due to LV systolic dysfunction ("pump failure") and the mechanical complications resulting from the infarction (**Figure 16-10**).

Figure 16-10

MANAGEMENT OF MECHANICAL COMPLICATIONS OF ACUTE MYOCARDIAL INFARCTION

I. **HYPOTENSION**
   - Right Ventricular Infarction
     —Administer IV fluids to augment RV filling pressure.
     —Avoid diuretics and nitrates.
     —Add positive inotropic agents (e.g., dobutamine or dopamine) if low cardiac output persists.
     —Institute temporary pacing, if high grade AV block and hemodynamic compromise is present (AV sequential pacing may be required to restore atrial transport).

II. **HYPERTENSION**
   - Adequate analgesics and sedation to relieve pain and anxiety.
   - Nitroglycerin, especially if ongoing ischemic chest pain, LV failure; Nitroprusside–potential "coronary steal" effect.
   - Beta blockers, particularly useful if hyperadrenergic state.
   - Diuretics, if volume depletion not present.
   - ACE inhibitors/ARBs, particularly if high-risk groups (e.g., anterior MI, CHF, ejection fraction < 40%).
   - Calcium channel blockers (after the acute phase), if LV failure (ejection fraction < 40%) not present.

III. **PUMP FAILURE AND CARDIOGENIC SHOCK**
   - Initiate invasive hemodynamic monitoring (to keep MAP > 60 mmHg, CI (CO/BSA) > 2.2 L/min/m2, and PCWP ~ 14-18 mmHg)*.
   - Administer pharmacologic support–optimize LV filling pressure and cardiac output.
     —Diuretics (e.g., furosemide, bumetanide, torsemide) to reduce pulmonary capillary wedge pressure.
     —Inotropic drugs (e.g., dopamine, dobutamine, or milrinone) to improve contractility.
     —Vasodilators (IV nitroglycerin, nitroprusside, and ACE inhibitors/ARBs (if ACE inhibitor intolerant [e.g., cough]), or ARNI [if not hypotensive]) to reduce preload and afterload.
   - Assure adequate ventilation and oxygenation.
   - Correct metabolic abnormalities.
   - Control tachy- and brady-arrhythmias.
   - Initiate mechanical circulatory assistance.
     —Intra-aortic balloon pump (IABP), percutaneous left ventricular assist device (LVAD), or extracorporeal membrane oxygenation (ECMO)-bridge to surgery.
   - Identify surgically correctable mechanical complications (ventricular septal rupture, acute mitral regurgitation, LV aneurysm).
   - Primary ("direct") percutaneous transluminal coronary angioplasty (PTCA)/stenting within initial hours of acute MI.

---

*Note: There is little evidence that the routine use of PA catheters in CHF patients improves clinical outcomes. Invasive hemodynamic monitoring, however, can be useful in acutely ill patients with decompensated CHF who have persistent symptoms despite standard therapies, whose fluid status or perfusion is uncertain, and in whom the measurements obtained are expected to guide therapy or influence management decisions.

Left Ventricular (LV) Systolic Dysfunction

Patients with an acute MI may come to medical attention with worsening heart failure, proportionate to the extent of myocardial necrosis, but exacerbated by preexisting dysfunction and ongoing ischemia. In general, damage to ≥25% of the myocardium results in LV systolic dysfunction. In patients with massive LV systolic dysfunction (i.e., damage to ≥40% of the myocardium), shock may occur. Four subgroups of patients with acute MI have been classified from low (*Class I*) to high (*Class IV*) mortality risk on the degree of LV systolic dysfunction by clinical examination (so-called *Killip classification*) (**Figure 16-11**). The therapy of the patient with an acute MI and resultant LV systolic dysfunction depends on the

Figure 16-11

KILLIP CLASSIFICATION OF ACUTE MYOCARDIAL INFARCTION

CLASS	CLINICAL EVIDENCE OF LV DYSFUNCTION	MORTALITY
I	No heart failure (uncomplicated) Absence of S3 gallop and pulmonary rales.	3–5%
II	Mild to moderate heart failure. Mild to moderate orthopnea. S3 gallop Bibasilar rales confined to ≤ 50% of both lung fields. Radiographic evidence of pulmonary venous congestion.	6–10%
III	Pulmonary edema. Severe respiratory distress. Rales heard over >50% of both lung fields. Radiographic evidence of interstitial and alveolar pulmonary edema	20–30%
IV	Cardiogenic shock Hypotension (systolic BP <90 mmHg) Tachycardia Signs of diminished peripheral perfusion: • Skin—cold, clammy, cyanotic. • CNS—mental confusion, agitation, obtundation. • Kidney—oliguria	> 80%

extent of such dysfunction. In most patients with symptoms and signs of Class II LV systolic dysfunction, CHF is transient, and usually responds to bed rest, salt restriction, and medical therapy, i.e., IV nitroglycerin, diuretics, ACE inhibitors, or angiotensin receptor blockers, and beta blockers.

In patients with more severe CHF unresponsive to medical therapy, as well as in those with pulmonary edema, hypotension, or evidence of systemic hypoperfusion, invasive hemodynamic monitoring may be necessary. Such measures include the Swan-Ganz catheter, along with vasopressors, inotropes, insertion of an IABP or percutaneous left ventricular assist device (LVAD), transthoracic or transesophageal echo and/or cardiac catheterization (with emergency PCI or even CABG) looking for a potentially correctable cause (e.g., acute MR, VSD). The therapeutic interventions used in the different hemodynamic subsets are listed in **Figure 16-12**.

Note: An increasingly recognized condition mimicking acute MI that causes acute reversible balloon-like LV systolic dysfunction, typically in the absence of obstructive CAD, is *stress cardiomyopathy*, also called *takotsubo cardiomyopathy, transient LV apical ballooning*, and *broken heart syndrome*. This disorder is often precipitated by sudden emotional or physical stress and occurs primarily in postmenopausal women. Despite the frequent occurrence of CHF or even cardiogenic shock, most patients recover completely within 1–4 weeks, and recurrence is rare.

Right Ventricular Infarction

The right coronary artery supplies blood to both the inferior wall of the LV and the RV wall.

Treatment should be directed at rapidly reperfusing the occluded coronary artery (via thrombolytic therapy, or direct PCI, particularly in high-risk patients with severe RV infarction). Patients should also receive volume expansion (i.e., saline infusions) directed toward increasing left heart filling so that cardiac output and arterial BP are restored to levels that sustain systemic perfusion. Inotropic therapy (e.g., dobutamine or dopamine) may also be required when hypoperfusion persists, to stimulate RV contractility.

It is important to keep in mind that nitrates, morphine, and/or diuretics can aggravate the condition by causing preload reduction and hypotension. In fact, if a patient with inferior MI develops profound hypotension upon initiation of these agents (especially nitroglycerin), the practitioner should strongly consider the diagnosis of right ventricular infarction. Patients with RV infarction have a stiff, noncompliant ventricle that depends on high filling pressures; thus, these patients may not tolerate the reduction in preload or venodilation induced by nitrates, morphine, and/or diuretics. Since a high venous filling pressure is required, if the elevated JVP is misconstrued to represent CHF (and diuretics and/or nitrates administered), there may be further compromise in the patient's clinical condition.

Figure 16-12

THERAPEUTIC INTERVENTION IN ACUTE
MYOCARDIAL INFARCTION

HEMODYNAMIC SUBSET	INTERVENTION
Normal	Aspirin and/or clopidogrel (if aspirin contra-indicated), ticagrelor, or prasugrel (if PCI planned); heparin or enoxaparin; nitrates (except in patients with suspected RV infarction and hypotension); beta blockers (if not contraindicated)*; thrombolytic therapy or percutaneous coronary intervention (PCI) if within 6–12 hrs of symptoms and onset of ST segment elevation MI; GP IIb/IIIa platelet receptor antagonists are given to high risk patients with unstable angina or non ST elevation MI, and patients undergoing PCI. Bivalirudin (if PCI planned) and fondaparinux (if no PCI planned) may be acceptable alternatives to heparin or enoxaparin.
Hyperdynamic state	Beta-blockers, then normal subset protocol.
Hypoperfusion (due to hypovolemia)	Fluid challenge, then normal subset protocol.
Congestive heart failure	Diuretic + ACE inhibitor/ARB + beta-blocker* + aldosterone blocker (eplerenone).
Cardiogenic shock	IV nitroglycerin, nitroprusside, dopamine, dobutamine, diuretic, circulatory assistance (IABP, LVAD), angioplasty/stenting or surgical revascularization and/or correction of mechanical complication (e.g., acute VSD, papillary muscle rupture).

IABP = intraaortic balloon pump, LVAD = left ventricular assist device (e.g., TandemHeart, Impella).
*Note: Early (<24 hr) use of IV beta blockers may increase risk of cardiogenic shock and should be avoided in patients with signs of CHF, evidence of low output state, or other risk factors, e.g., age > 70 yrs, systolic BP < 120 mmHg, sinus tachycardia > 110/min., heart rate < 60/min. or delayed presentation after symptom onset. In the absence of contraindications, oral beta blockers should be continued for up to 3 years after uncomplicated MI, and indefinitely in patients with LV systolic dysfunction.

Pericarditis

Pericarditis is a common complication of acute ST segment elevation MI. The correct identification of pericarditis as the cause of recurrent chest pain is important, since treatment with aspirin is indicated. Failure to recognize pericarditis may lead to the erroneous diagnosis of recurrent ischemic chest pain with resultant inappropriate use of anticoagulants, nitrates, beta blockers or coronary angiography. Anticoagulation therapy potentially could cause tamponade in the presence of pericarditis and therefore should not be used unless there is a compelling indication. Often, no treatment is required, but aspirin will usually relieve the pain. Nonsteroidal antiinflammatory agents and steroids are generally avoided since they may inhibit healing of the infarct.

Dressler's (post-MI) syndrome is an immunologic phenomenon characterized by pericardial pain, generalized malaise, fever, elevated white blood cell count and erythrocyte sedimentation rate, and pericardial effusion. It occurs several weeks to months after MI. As in acute pericarditis, aspirin should be given as primary therapy, while steroids and nonsteroidal antiinflammatory agents should be avoided if possible until at least one month has elapsed since MI.

SECONDARY PREVENTION: PHARMACOLOGIC THERAPY, RISK FACTOR MODIFICATION, AND CARDIAC REHABILITATION

The goals of therapy for patients with acute MI are to limit infarct size, increase myocardial oxygen supply, decrease myocardial oxygen demand, promote electrical stability, and prevent or manage mechanical complications. Early recognition and appropriate treatment of these electrical and mechanical complications are essential to reduce morbidity and mortality.

In general, the foundation of care in acute coronary syndromes has undergone remarkable evolution over the past several years. Recent data from numerous well-designed clinical trials have shed considerable light on the optimal therapeutic approach (**Figure 16-13**). An overall summary of beneficial and non-beneficial measures in the acute and long-term treatment of MI is presented in **Figure 16-14**. In addition to aggressive reperfusion strategies (e.g., thrombolytic agents, "direct" PCI), aimed at rapid and complete restoration of coronary blood flow through the infarct-related artery, adjunctive pharmacologic therapies have been shown to improve survival and reduce the incidence of re-infarction. These adjunctive therapies include beta blockers, aspirin, P2Y12 inhibitors, statins, heparin, warfarin, ACE inhibitors/ARBs, and aldosterone blockers, particularly in patients with diminished LV function (ejection fraction <40%).

The ischemic and thrombotic benefit but increased bleeding risk of ticagrelor and prasugrel over clopidogrel (particularly the latter in patients who have a prior stroke or TIA, are >75 years of age, or weigh <60 kg), the potentially harmful effects of the short-acting dihydropyridine calcium channel blockers (e.g., nife-

Figure 16-13

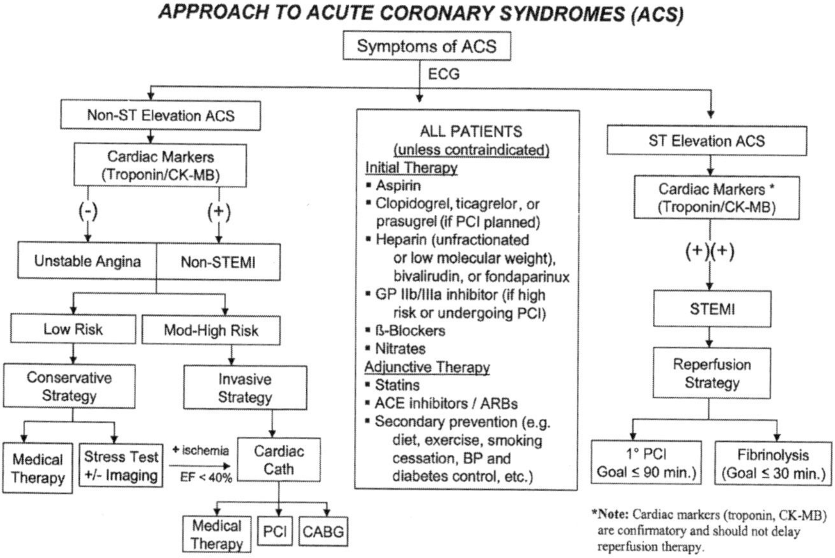

APPROACH TO ACUTE CORONARY SYNDROMES (ACS)

Note: In non-ST elevation ACS (unstable angina, nonSTEMI) an early invasive strategy (cath and possible revascularization) is advised in high risk patients. Primary PCI is preferred over fibrinolysis in STEMI patients if it is available within 90 minutes (120 minutes if transferring to a PCI-capable hospital) Unless contraindicated, the more potent P2Y12 inhibitors ticagrelor and prasugrel (at the time of PCI) are preferred over clopidogrel in ACS, except in STEMI patients undergoing fibrinolysis, or in those at high risk of bleeding.

---

dipine), the limited role of the rate-slowing non-dihydropyridine calcium channel blockers (e.g., diltiazem, verapamil) in the setting of non ST elevation MI and intact LV function, the lack of mortality benefit of routine magnesium in a large clinical "megatrial", the lack of benefit of routine late PCI of an occluded infarct-related artery in stable patients days to weeks after MI and the trend toward a higher incidence of cardiovascular events within the first year of initiation of hormone (estrogen/progesterone) replacement therapy in older postmenopausal women, the potentially detrimental effects of routine prophylactic lidocaine, the "proarrhythmic" effects of empiric class I antiarrhythmic agents, and the survival advantage of ICD therapy in patients 40 days or more post-MI who have an LV ejection fraction of 30% or less, have also been noted.

In more recent times, a new wave of clot-specific thrombolytics (e.g., alteplase [t-PA], reteplase [r-PA], tenecteplase [TNK-tPA]), antithrombotics (e.g., UFH, enoxaparin, fondaparinux, bivalirudin), and antiplatelet agents (e.g., GP IIb/IIIa blockers, clopidogrel, prasugrel, ticagrelor, vorapaxar) have come into the

Figure 16-14

MODERN TREATMENT OF ACUTE MYOCARDIAL INFARCTION

	ACUTE	LONG-TERM
Significant benefit	• Reperfusion therapy (if ST elevation MI) —Thrombolytic agents (e.g., TPA, rPA, TNK-TPA, SK) —Primary PCI, "rescue" PCI (if thrombolysis fails), or routine early PCI (after successful fibrinolysis) in PCI-capable centers • Aspirin (chewed, oral) and/or clopidogrel, ticagrelor, or prasugrel (with PCI). • GP IIb/IIIa antagonists–if non STEMI or in high risk patients (e.g., large thrombus burden) undergoing PCI • Heparin —IV unfractionated with PCI or fibrin selective thrombolytic agents (e.g., TPA, rPA, TNK-TPA) to maintain coronary patency • IV unfractionated or Sub Q low molecular weight heparin (e.g., enoxaparin [Lovenox], dalteparin [Fragmin]), in anterior MI to reduce risk of mural thrombus and systemic embolization. Recent trials support use of enoxaparin or fondaparinux in the setting of thrombolysis. —Low dose Sub Q to prevent deep venous thrombosis and pulmonary embolism (especially if elderly, obesity, congestive heart failure or prolonged immobilization)	• Aspirin and/or clopidogrel, prasugrel, or ticagrelor, if aspirin intolerant. Both for non STEMI/STEMI and PCI. • Beta blockers —especially high-risk patient with large or anterior MI and recurrent ischemia, LV dysfunction or complex ventricular ectopy • ACE inhibitors (or ARBs or ARNI) —if asymptomatic patient with LV ejection fraction < 40% or symptomatic heart failure • Risk factor modification —Smoking cessation; BP, lipid, and glucose control; treatment of obesity; and moderate physical activity —HMG CoA reductase inhibitors ("statins") to reduce LDL cholesterol > 50%, if tolerated • Warfarin —Following IV heparin if large anterior MI, apical dyskinesis, LV thrombus or systemic embolization • Rate-limiting calcium channel blockers (diltiazem, verapamil) —Following non STEMI with preserved LV function ast 40 days post-MI

90

| **Significant benefit** | • Beta blockers (IV, oral), if no contraindication
　—with or without thrombolysis
• ACE inhibitors (oral)
　—especially large anterior MI without hypotension
• Acute nitrates
　—If ischemic chest pain, LV dysfunction, or hypertension is present
• IABP
　—To enhance thrombolytic efficacy, reduce reocclusion after PCI, or as "bridge" to surgery
• Emergency CABG
　—If failed reperfusion (PCI), left main or severe 3 vessel CAD. | • Aldosterone blocker (eplerenone)
　—in patients with LV systolic dysfunction and CHF receiving standard therapy (e.g., beta blockers and ACE inhibitors/ARBs)
• Implantable cardioverter-defibrillator in patients with VT/VF or EF ≤ 30% at least 40 days post-MI |
| **Doubtful efficacy or Potentially harmful** | • Calcium channel blockers
　—Especially immediate-release dihydropyridines
• Routine prophylactic lidocaine (decreases risk of primary VF but also increases risk of fatal asystolic events) is no longer recommended
　—Reserved for sustained/ symptomatic ventricular tachycardia, ventricular fibrillation, or "complex" (frequent, multifocal) PVCs
• Nitrates for RV MI (preload dependent)
• Magnesium sulfate
　—Not recommended routinely, however, may be beneficial for post-infarction ventricular arrhythmias and torsades de pointes, especially if hypomagnesemia is present.
• Beta blockers in cocaine-induced MI (may potentiate coronary spasm)
• Fibrinolytics in unstable angina/non STEMI | • Class I antiarrhythmic agents (proarrhythmic effect-torsades de pointes)
• Calcium channel blockers
　—If severe LV dysfunction or heart failure is present
• Hormone therapy during first year in older postmenopausal women
• Nitrates within 24 – 48 hours of sildenafil (Viagra), vardenafil (Levitra), or tadalafil (Cialis).
• Late PCI of an occluded infarct-related artery in stable patients days to weeks after MI
• NSAIDs, nonselective or COX-2 selective |

limelight. The appropriate choices of treatment is dictated the type, location and severity of MI, the extent of accompanying ischemia, the degree of LV dysfunction, and the presence of supraventricular and ventricular arrhythmias and conduction disturbances, mural thrombus formation, and other associated complications.

In this era of fascination with new technologies and innovative treatment strategies, the practitioner must not neglect the importance of secondary prevention measures including risk factor modification. These risk factor modifications include smoking cessation, proper diet, lipid-lowering therapy, hypertension and diabetes control, weight reduction (if appropriate), stress management techniques, supervised exercise, and cardiac rehabilitation. These measures aim to halt the progression or enhance the regression of atherosclerotic cardiovascular disease, as part of the contemporary management scheme. In terms of cholesterol lowering, patients should be treated with high dose statins as tolerated. In addition to lowering LDL-cholesterol, early administration of high dose HMG CoA reductase inhibitors ("statins") have been shown to be beneficial in reducing vascular inflammation, improving endothelial function, stabilizing impending plaque rupture, and reducing CAD events and mortality (so-called "pleiotropic effects"). Serum markers of inflammation e.g., high sensitivity C-reactive protein (CRP) levels may help to identify those patients at risk who will benefit most from statin therapy (<1 mg/L = low risk, $1–3$ mg/L = intermediate risk, >3 mg/L = high risk). Although recent studies suggest an association between improved clinical outcomes and lower CRP levels after statin treatment, there is no definitive evidence that lower CRP levels *per se* prevent vascular events. While optimal risk reduction strategies are of paramount importance, it must be realized that an optimistic attitude on the part of the practitioner and the entire health-care team from the outset, along with continued reassurance as to the patient's ultimate recovery and return to normal activities, are essential requisites to an improved quality of life and overall clinical outcome.

Chapter 17.   Heart Failure

Heart failure is a complex clinical syndrome resulting from a structural or functional abnormality that impairs the ability of the ventricles to eject or fill with blood. It is commonly termed "congestive" heart failure (CHF), since signs and symptoms of increased pulmonary and/or systemic venous pressure are often prominent. Although CHF is common, it is not a specific diagnosis in and of itself, but rather is the result of some underlying cardiac or occasionally noncardiac disorder. This chapter will review the practical clinical approach to pharmacologic treatment of the patient who presents with *chronic* or *acute* heart failure with LV *systolic* (reduced EF) or *diastolic* (preserved EF) *dysfunction*.

In general, CHF can be divided into two main categories: *systolic dysfunction* (due to reduced LV contractility), which is most common, and *diastolic dysfunction* (due to impaired LV relaxation and filling).

Left Ventricular Systolic Dysfunction

It is estimated that more than 5 million Americans have CHF, and approximately 500,000 new cases are diagnosed each year. CHF due to LV systolic dysfunction is a common complication of many types of heart disease, e.g.:

- CAD with ischemic LV damage (i.e., acute MI, acute MR/VSD, LV aneurysm, "ischemic cardiomyopathy")
- Chronic systemic arterial hypertension
- Dilated cardiomyopathy
- Valvular heart disease with its pressure (e.g., AS) and/or volume (e.g., MR, AR) overloading of the heart.

In fact, CHF is the most frequently used (and most expensive) cardiovascular hospital diagnosis-related group (DRG) discharge diagnosis in the United States today. CAD is the underlying cause of CHF in ~2/3 of patients with LV systolic dysfunction. The remainder have nonischemic causes e.g., hypertension, valvular heart disease, myocardial toxins (i.e., alcohol or doxorubicin), myocarditis, or no identifiable cause, e.g., idiopathic dilated cardiomyopathy.

93

Left Ventricular Diastolic Dysfunction

LV diastolic dysfunction is usually associated with *LV hypertrophy* (due to hypertension, valvular AS or HOCM), CAD (ischemia, acute MI), small vessel disease (e.g., diabetes mellitus), *restrictive cardiomyopathy* (e.g., amyloidosis, sarcoidosis, hemochromatosis, scleroderma), or the aging process. Although LV contractility is normal, there is impaired LV relaxation and filling to such an extent that heart failure and even acute ("flash") pulmonary edema may result (e.g., with the onset of rapid atrial fibrillation). Diastolic dysfunction is responsible for approximately 50% of all heart failure episodes, particularly in patients with associated CAD and/or hypertension. Its incidence increases with age and is higher in women than in men.

Treatment of Chronic Heart Failure

Effective management of CHF focuses on searching for and correcting the predisposing risk factors and underlying cause, if possible. These include identifying and treating CAD, hypertension, diabetes mellitus, dyslipidemia, anemia, or thyroid disease; repairing or replacing a significantly regurgitant or stenotic heart valve; restoring blood flow to an obstructed coronary artery (by PCI or CABG); correcting a persistently fast heart rate or restoring sinus rhythm (as in atrial fibrillation, SVT); eliminating alcohol intake (alcohol may cause a cardiomyopathy); and avoiding drugs (if possible) that may aggravate the condition. Such drugs include NSAIDs, steroids, and thiazolidinediones (which cause fluid retention), and the anticancer drug doxorubicin, which causes cardiomyopathy. Many types of medications exist to help reduce the symptoms of systolic CHF and potentially prolong life. In contrast to systolic dysfunction, no medications are approved yet to reduce mortality in patients with diastolic dysfunction.

The "ABCs" of the pharmacologic treatment of systolic LV dysfunction include:

A: ACE inhibitors e.g., captopril (Capoten), enalapril (Vasotec), lisinopril (Zestril, Prinivil), ramipril (Altace), fosinopril (Monopril), quinapril (Accupril) benazepril (Lotensin), trandolapril (Mavik). These drugs help reduce symptoms and increase survival, in all patients with LV EF < 40% and/or

Angiotensin II receptor-blockers (ARBs), e.g., losartan (Cozaar), irbesartan (Avapro), candesartan (Atacand), valsartan (Diovan), olmesartan (Benicar), telmisartan (Micardis), eprosartan (Teveten) especially if intolerant to side effects of ACE inhibitors (e.g., cough, angioneurotic edema)

Angiotensin receptor neprilysin inhibitor (ARNI), e.g., valsartan/sacubitril (Entresto), in place of ACE inhibitor or ARB, to reduce mortality and hospitalization.

Aldosterone antagonists, e.g., spironolactone (Aldactone), in patients with advanced CHF, and eplerenone (Inspra), in post-MI patients with CHF. These drugs reduce mortality, but may cause hyperkalemia (especially if combined with ACE inhibitors/ARBs).

B: Beta blockers, e.g., carvedilol (Coreg, Coreg-CR), long-acting metroprolol succinate (Toprol-XL), bisoprolol (Zebeta), as tolerated. These drugs help reduce symptoms and increase survival (starting with a low dose and building up gradually over a period of weeks).

B-type or Brain Natriuretic Peptide i.e., IV nesiritide (Natrecor), for acutely decompensated CHF

C: Combination therapy e.g., hydralazine (Apresoline), a pure arterial vasodilator, and nitrates, a venodilating agent, should also be considered if intolerant to ACE inhibitors or ARBs (particularly if renal insufficiency or hyperkalemia are limiting factors), or in African-Americans.

Coumadin (warfarin), especially if severe dilated cardiomyopathy, atrial fibrillation, mechanical heart valves, or previous history of systemic or pulmonary embolism are present.

Cardiac Inotropes i.e., IV sympathomimetic amines e.g., dopamine (Intropin), dobutamine (Dobutrex), and phosphodiesterase inhibitors e.g., milrinone (Primacor), for severe and/or end-stage CHF

D: Diuretics, help reduce symptoms and decrease hospitalization rates. The goal is to achieve a "dry weight" as determined by reducing the elevated JVP and the abnormal abdominojugular reflux, along with other signs of fluid retention (e.g., rales, peripheral edema). A simple bedside scale with routine recording of weight is a helpful tool to determine diuretic response. *Avoid overly vigorous diuresis.* An excessive reduction of blood volume may actually reduce cardiac output, interfere with renal function, and produce profound weakness and lethargy. Exercise caution when using diuretics in patients with "restrictive filling" hemodynamics (e.g., HOCM, constrictive pericarditis). Remember to avoid diuretics (and nitrates) in patients with RV infarction (since they decrease preload, while the stiff RV needs higher intraventricular pressure to function).

Digoxin (Lanoxin), improves symptoms and decreases hospitalization rates (but has no survival benefit). It may be beneficial when rapid atrial fibrillation is present. (**Note:** It is important to avoid a low potassium level. Hypokalemia can precipitate potentially dangerous ventricular arrhythmias, particularly in patients who are receiving digoxin. You should lower digoxin dose when taking verapamil, quinidine, amiodarone and dronedarone. These drugs raise digoxin levels.)

Diet (restrict sodium and limit fluid intake)—to reduce fluid accumulation (edema) in the lungs, liver, abdomen and legs. Abstain from alcohol (because of its myocardial depressant effects).

Diuretics may be more effective, however, on the days when there is less physical activity. Many patients have little or no diuretic response during busy weekdays, but on a quiet, more restful weekend have a prompt and/or significant response (due to increased preload to the heart when the patient is at rest that improves cardiac output and renal perfusion). Thiazides, e.g., hydrochlorothiazide (HydroDIURIL), chlorothiazide (Diuril), chlorthalidone (Hygroton), and indapamide (Lozol), are standard therapy for chronic CHF (without renal insufficiency) when edema is mild to modest. Effectiveness is limited by intense proximal tubular reabsorption of sodium in more advanced stages of CHF (thiazides work in the distal tubule). With more advanced degrees of CHF (or when renal insufficiency is present, i.e., creatinine >2 mg/dL) the stronger loop diuretics and/or combinations of diuretics may be needed. Such drugs may include thiazide or thiazide-like agent metolazone (Zaroxolyn) and an intravenous loop diuretic e.g., furosemide (Lasix), bumetanide (Bumex), torsemide (Demadex). Torsemide and bumetanide have greater bioavailability and may be considered in patients with significant right-sided CHF, where absorption of furosemide is frequently unpredictable. A short course of IV diuretics may improve absorption and effectiveness of oral agents by helping to reduce gut edema. Spironolactone (Aldactone), a potassium-sparing diuretic (when added to an ACE inhibitor and a loop diuretic, with or without digoxin) has been shown to improve CHF symptoms and reduce mortality rates (spironolactone is an aldosterone antagonist that counteracts the adverse effects of excess aldosterone on ventricular remodeling). A newer aldosterone antagonist, eplerenone (Inspra), also appears effective in preventing LV remodeling and has been shown to improve survival in post-MI patients with CHF.

Even if the patient has responded favorably to a diuretic, treatment with an ACE inhibitor (and/or ARB) and a beta blocker should be initiated and maintained unless these drugs are not tolerated or their use is contraindicated. Vasodilators are important treatment in patients with CHF. *ACE inhibitors are clearly the vasodilator of choice. ACE inhibitors, along with beta blockers and aldosterone antagonists, prolong life, whereas loop and thiazide diuretics as well as digoxin just relieve symptoms.*

The combination of a pure *arterial vasodilator* (e.g., *hydralazine* [Apresoline]) and a strong *venodilating agent* (e.g., *nitrates*) can reduce afterload, improve forward flow (cardiac output), decrease filling pressure (preload), improve congestive symptoms, and has been shown to reduce mortality. This combination was used for many years in patients with CHF before the advent of ACE inhibitors. Although this potent vasodilator pair improves survival, studies have shown that ACE inhibitors do so to an even greater extent. In patients who cannot tolerate ACE inhibitors (or ARBs), however, or when symptoms persist despite aggressive therapy with ACE inhibitors and diuretics, the combination of hydralazine and nitrates remains a viable option. Of note, the combination of isosorbide dinitrate (a nitric oxide donor) and hydralazine (an antioxidant that inhibits destruction of nitric oxide) (BiDil) has been shown to be particularly beneficial in African-Americans with CHF (who may have a less active renin-angiotensin system and a lower bioavailability of nitric oxide).

Therapy with digoxin may be initiated at any time to reduce symptoms or to slow the ventricular response in patients with rapid atrial fibrillation. It may seem paradoxical that beta blockers can exacerbate or worsen CHF (negative inotropic effect) and are now considered first-line treatment for CHF, but both are true. There is mounting clinical evidence that if stable patients are initiated on low doses of a beta blocker e.g., carvedilol, long-acting metoprolol succinate (not short-acting tartrate), or bisoprolol (added to standard CHF therapy) with gradual upward titration, they may derive significant benefit. The mechanism of this benefit may relate to blunting of the cardiotoxic effects of excess circulating catecholamines and improvement in LV size and shape (so-called reverse-remodeling). Following several weeks of therapy, beta blockers have been consistently shown to increase ejection fraction by 5 to 10 points (e.g., from an ejection fraction of 20% to 25–30%). Furthermore, data suggest that beta blockers slow the progression of CHF, reduce hospitalization and the need for adjustments of other CHF medications and heart transplantation, and they reduce mortality.

Of note, a novel heart rate lowering agent, ivabradine (Corlanor), that acts by selectively inhibiting the I_f ("funny") current in the sinoatrial node, has recently been approved as add-on therapy to reduce the risk of hospitalization (but not mortality) for worsening heart failure in patients with chronic stable, symptomatic CHF with reduced ejection fraction $\leq 35\%$, who are in sinus rhythm with a resting heart rate ≥ 70 beats per minute, and who are on maximum tolerated doses of beta blockers or have a contraindication to their use. Unlike beta blockers, ivabradine has no effect on myocardial contractility (i.e., no negative inotropic effect).

Worthy of mention, a new class of drug called angiotensin receptor neprilysin inhibitor (ARNI), combines an ARB (valsartan) with a neprilysin inhibitor (sacubitril) and blocks both the angiotensin (ATI) receptor and the enzymatic breakdown of endogenous natriuretic and vasodilatory peptides. This novel combination drug (Entresto) has been shown to be more effective than an ACE inhibitor (enalapril) in reducing cardiovascular mortality and hospitalization and holds promise as a first line treatment of CHF.

Selected patients with severe CHF also may benefit symptomatically from ultrafiltration (which reduces fluid overload) and the periodic IV infusion of inotropic agents, such as:

- the sympathomimetic amines including dopamine (Intropin) (which at low dosages stimulates dopaminergic receptors in the renal vascular bed causing increased renal blood flow which facilitates diuresis, and at moderate doses increases inotropy by stimulating cardiac β-1 receptors
- dobutamine (Dobutrex), a synthetic analog of dopamine that preferentially stimulates β-1 receptors in addition to β-2 and α receptors
- milrinone (Primacor), a phosphodiesterase-3 inhibitor, which increases calcium uptake, myocardial contractility, stroke volume, ejection fraction and sinus rate, while decreasing peripheral resistance (and thus act as an "inotropic dilator")

Dobutamine must be used with caution in patients with systolic blood pressure less than 100 mmHg because it can worsen hypotension. Since dobutamine and milrinone may adversely affect survival (due to increased incidence of ventricular tachyarrhythmias), these agents should be reserved for short-term administration in patients with end-stage CHF refractory to conventional therapy.

Nitroprusside (Nipride) remains the primary intravenous vasodilator for the hospitalized CHF patient (especially in the setting of hypertension). This balanced venous and arterial dilator reduces pulmonary and systemic vascular resistance with improved hemodynamics and enhanced diuresis. Side effects include excess hypotension, paradoxical oxygen desaturation due to AV shunting, coronary steal, and cyanide toxicity. IV *nesiritide* (Natrecor), a genetically engineered recombinant form of human BNP approved for the treatment of acute decompensated CHF, acts as a potent vasodilator and natriuretic factor that reduces ventricular filling pressure, enhances diuresis, and improves cardiac output. Nesiritide has not been shown to provide a clear clinical benefit over standard therapy, however, and its use is not routinely recommended.

In some situations, however, the heart becomes so weak that conventional medical treatment has little impact. In selected patients with a widened QRS complex, resynchronization therapy with *biventricular pacing* appears to induce an improvement in symptoms and survival. *Left ventricular assist devices* and *heart transplantation* may need to be considered for those patients with end-stage CHF refractory to all other therapeutic measures. Contraindications to heart transplantation include old age, pulmonary hypertension, infection (including HIV), co-morbid conditions that significantly limit life expectancy, unresolved alcohol and/or drug abuse, and a noncompliant patient.

When using potent diuretics, normal serum potassium (and magnesium) levels need to be carefully maintained. Taking potassium-sparing diuretics (e.g., spironolactone), potassium supplements, eating potassium-rich foods, and/or monitoring serum potassium levels are precautionary measures. Keep in mind that hyperkalemia may result when potassium-sparing diuretics and/or supplements are administered to patients taking ACE inhibitors (which can cause hyperkalemia) and in patients with renal insufficiency, particularly if diabetic.

It is important to emphasize that patients who are symptomatic with dyspnea at rest or who are hemodynamically unstable should not be started on beta blocker therapy. Patients receiving beta blocker therapy may need a dose reduction or discontinuance if clinically significant cardiac decompensation develops. Decompensation may, however, respond to an increase in diuretic dose without requiring beta blocker withdrawal. The clinician should always try to ascertain if there is a history of high sodium and fluid intake or medication noncompliance when decompensation occurs. One of the most common causes of an acute exacerbation of CHF is inadvertent or inappropriate reduction in therapy. This may occur through noncompliance on the part of the patient with compensated CHF and mild symptoms or through changes in medications made by other practitioners.

In the "real world", patients often discontinue medication or fail to renew their prescriptions ("I ran out of my pills") because they are taking too many drugs, too many each day, are spending too much money, and have too many side effects. Whenever possible, therefore, try to keep it simple. Prescribe long-acting and/or combination preparations (if possible). Keep in mind that the cost of multiple drug therapy is an extremely important concern to patients, particularly those who are retired, or on disability programs with fixed incomes and limited insurance coverage (**Figure 17-1**).

Figure 17-1

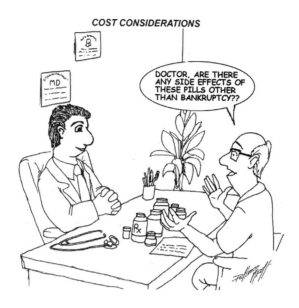

Ambulatory patients with CHF should adhere to a restricted sodium diet. Limiting total fluid intake to 1500–2000 ml/day (or less if hyponatremia is present) is a reasonable guideline for most patients with CHF. Some patients may need to be overdiuresed in order to prevent congestive symptoms.

The "ABCs" of treating diastolic dysfunction:

A: Avoid digoxin (Lanoxin), unless systolic LV dysfunction and/or rapid atrial fibrillation is also present (digoxin acts by increasing systolic contractility, which is not needed in diastolic dysfunction). Especially avoid digoxin in HOCM, where an increased LV contractility can worsen the outflow tract gradient.

ACE inhibitors (effect on ventricular remodeling), e.g., captopril (Capoten), enalapril (Vasotec), lisinopril (Zestril, Prinivil), ramipril (Altace), fosinopril (Monopril), quinapril (Accupril). **Note: ARBs** may be used if ACE intolerant.

Aldosterone antagonists, e.g., spironolactone (Aldactone), may reduce hospitalization for CHF and cardiovascular mortality (controversial)

B: Beta blockers, e.g., propranolol (Inderal), metoprolol (Lopressor, Toprol-XL), atenolol (Tenormin), nadolol (Corgard), acebutolol (Sectral). Beta blockers and calcium channel blockers (particularly verapamil and diltiazem) enhance diastolic relaxation (in addition to decreasing systolic contractility) (especially in hypertrophic cardiomyopathy) and decrease heart rate, which in turn increases diastolic filling time (a key goal in patients with CHF and LV hypertrophy).

C: Calcium channel blockers, e.g., dihydropyridines (nifedipine [Procardia, Adalat], amlodipine [Norvasc], felodipine [Plendil], isradipine [DynaCirc], nisoldipine [Sular]), and nondihydropyridines (verapamil [Isoptin, Calan, Verelan], and diltiazem [Cardizem, Tiazac, Dilacor]).

D: Diuretics, e.g., furosemide (Lasix), bumetanide (Bumex), torsemide (Demadex) for symptoms of fluid overload, to reduce the congestive state. (**Note:** Monitor diuretic effects carefully since excessive administration may result in a drop in cardiac output, hypotension and prerenal azotemia.)

Diet (low sodium)

When treating patients with diastolic dysfunction, it is important to keep in mind the importance of correcting the underlying remediable causes and exacerbating factors, e.g., by:

- Valve replacement in aortic stenosis
- Preventing tachycardia (with beta blockers, calcium channel blockers, catheter ablation and pacing) and maintaining atrial contraction (by electrical or pharmacologic cardioversion)
- Controlling hypertension (with antihypertensive agents)
- Treating myocardial ischemia (with nitrates, beta blockers, calcium channel blockers, PCI, or CABG) that may impair LV relaxation.

Treatment of Acute Heart Failure and Pulmonary Edema

Acute heart failure may develop suddenly in a previously asymptomatic patient (e.g., with an ACS, a hypertensive crisis, or acute aortic regurgitation (AR)/mitral regurgitation (MR)), or it may complicate chronic compensated CHF following a precipitating event (e.g., dietary indiscretion, medication noncompliance, intercurrent illness or infection, arrhythmias, e.g., rapid atrial fibrillation or VT, anemia, thyroid disease, alcohol, or drugs, e.g., NSAIDs, steroids, thiazolidinediones) and toxins (e.g., cocaine, anthracyclines). The patient's volume status (wet vs. dry) and adequacy of tissue perfusion (cold vs. warm) should be assessed.

Patients presenting with acute pulmonary edema require immediate stabilization. The goal of therapy is to improve oxygenation and reduce elevated left heart filling pressure. The patient should be placed in a sitting position with legs dangling over the side of the bed to reduce venous return and ease breathing. Supplemental oxygen should be delivered by face mask (to maintain O_2 sat > 90 %), and morphine sulfate given intravenously to reduce preload as well as patient anxiety (through its action on opiate receptors in the brain). Watch for respiratory depression. Loop diuretics (e.g., furosemide, bumetanide, torsemide) are administered intravenously (either as a bolus or continuous infusion), without delay, and in addition to their diuretic properties, also produce venodilation, thereby reducing LV preload. Vasodilators, e.g., nitroglycerin (sublingual and/or intravenous), or nesiritide, titrated by clinical and blood pressure response, reduce both preload and afterload and are especially useful in the presence of hypertension and myocardial ischemia. Intravenous nitroprusside (with careful monitoring) in patients with severe MR or AR, and inotropic drugs (e.g., dopamine, dobutamine, milrinone) may be considered for hemodynamic support. For patients with symptomatic hypotension and end-organ dysfunction (cardiogenic shock) despite IV vasoactive therapy, mechanical support (e.g., IABP, LVAD, extracorporeal membrane oxygenation [ECMO]) should be considered. The patient should be monitored by continuous pulse oximetry and if respiratory failure ensues, intubated and mechanical ventilation begun.

During resolution of the acute event, attention should be directed at identifying and treating the underlying cause.

Pearls:

- Unless contraindicated, patients with CHF with reduced ejection fraction should take an ACE inhibitor (or ARB) and a beta blocker to reduce mortality, and if volume overloaded, a diuretic to decrease symptoms.

- Addition of an aldosterone antagonist can reduce mortality and hospitalization for CHF.

- The combination of hydralazine and isosorbide dinitrate has been shown to reduce mortality and symptoms of CHF in African Americans.

- Digoxin can decrease symptoms and lower the rate of hospitalization for CHF, but does not reduce mortality.

- A new class of drug, ARNI, which combines an ARB with a neprilysin inhibitor, has been shown to be superior to an ACE inhibitor in reducing mortality and hospitalization for CHF.

- In patients with advanced CHF with reduced ejection fraction ≤ 35%, LBBB and a wide QRS complex ≥ 150 msec, device therapy with ICD and CRT (biventricular pacing) can improve symptoms and reduce hospitalization and mortality for CHF.

- There is little evidence that drug treatment improves clinical outcomes in patients with HFpEF (with the exception of an aldosterone antagonist [controversial]).

- Keep in mind the *mnemonic* "**LMNOP**" in the management of acute pulmonary edema.
  - **L**oop diuretics
  - **M**orphine
  - **N**itroglycerin
  - **O**xygen
  - Upright **P**osition

Chapter 18.   Systemic Arterial Hypertension

Hypertension is a powerful risk factor for acute MI, CHF, stroke, renal failure, aortic aneurysm and/or dissection. It is the most common disease-specific reason for practitioner visits in the United States today. According to updated guidelines issued by the American Heart Association, nearly half of the adults in the United States (~100 million) are now considered to have hypertension, redefined as a BP ≥ 130/80 mmHg (down from the previous standard of 140/90 mmHg), and up to three times as many African-Americans have an elevated BP than does the general population. It has also been reported that of the 70% of adults who are aware of their diagnosis, only one third to one half are being adequately treated.

The great majority (95%) of patients have no identifiable cause and are said to have essential or primary hypertension. Although the specific cause is unknown, familial patterns of primary hypertension are common. In addition, environmental factors e.g., obesity, alcohol consumption, sedentary lifestyle, salt intake, and psychogenic stress may play a role. If hypertension is unresponsive to medical therapy or hypertension is in an accelerated phase, you should evaluate the patient for the possibility of an underlying curable secondary cause.

This chapter will review the practical clinical approach to the patient with systemic arterial hypertension.

When an elevated BP reading is detected, it should be measured at least twice during two separate examinations after the initial screening. Transient elevation of BP caused by excitement or apprehension does not constitute hypertensive disease but may indicate a propensity toward its evolution. A progressive and linear relationship exists between increasing BP and cardiovascular risk, beginning at a BP of 115/75 mmHg and doubling with each increment of 20/10 mmHg. Defining a precise cutoff point at which BP is considered "high", therefore, is somewhat arbitrary. Although hypertension in adults has been traditionally defined as a BP ≥ 140/90 mmHg, recent clinical trial data have identified groups of patients at increased cardiovascular risk in whom BPs below this value may be associated with improved outcomes. Accordingly, recently revised guidelines now define a "normal BP" as a BP < 120/80 mmHg; an "elevated BP" (previously termed "prehypertension") as a BP 120-129/<80 mmHg; "stage 1 hypertension" as a BP 130-139/80-89 mmHg; and "stage 2 hypertension" as a BP ≥ 140/90 mmHg. A "hypertensive crisis" is defined as a severe elevation in BP (BP > 180/120 mmHg) with (hypertensive emergency) or without (hypertensive urgency) evidence of new or worsening target organ damage or dysfunction. (**Figure 18-1**).

Figure 18-1. Updated classification of BP for adults aged ≥ 18 years.

Figure 18-1

CLASSIFICATION OF BLOOD PRESSURE FOR ADULTS AGED ≥ 18 YEARS*

BP CATEGORY	SYSTOLIC BP, mmHg	DIASTOLIC BP, mmHG
Normal BP	< 120	< 80
Elevated BP	120-129	< 80
Stage 1 hypertension	130-139	80-89
Stage 2 hypertension	≥ 140	≥ 90
Hypertensive crisis** (emergency/urgency)	> 180	>120

*Note: Blood pressure (BP) is categorized as normal, elevated, and stage 1 or 2 hypertension, based on an average of ≥ 2 careful readings obtained on ≥ 2 occasions. Individuals with systolic BP and diastolic BP in 2 categories should be designated to the higher BP category.
**Hypertensive crises are divided into 2 types, emergencies or urgencies, based on the presence or absence of new or worsening target organ damage or dysfunction, respectively.

Adapted from Whelton PK, Carey RM, Aronow WS, et. al., ACC/AHA Guideline for the Prevention, Detection, Evaluation, and Management of High Blood Pressure in Adults; A Report of the American College of Cardiology/American Heart Association Task Force on Clinical Practice Guidelines. Hypertension, 2018.

Treatment of Hypertension

Currently, up to 30% of those with hypertension remain undiagnosed and only one third to one half of those known to have high blood pressure are adequately controlled. Institution of early antihypertensive therapy will not only prevent the development of hypertensive heart disease but will also reduce the morbidity and mortality from CAD, CHF, kidney disease and stroke.

Hypertension control begins with proper detection and diagnosis. There is both overdiagnosis e.g., *"white coat"* (office) *hypertension*, whereby the stress of visiting the practitioner may sometimes lead to falsely elevated BP readings, as well as underdiagnosis (due to lack of taking BP or poor BP technique). Proper diagnosis requires correct BP measurement techniques (automated vs manual [auscultatory]) and confirmation of high blood pressure with repeat measurements on at least two separate occasions before establishing a diagnosis and the need for treatment. Be aware of circumstances that temporarily raise blood pressure in the absence of disease (e.g., anxiety, rushing to make the appointment on time, bladder distention, recent cigarette smoking, alcohol or caffeine intake, improper technique, such as wrong cuff size).

In deciding if and when to treat your patient with hypertension, have him or her keep a log of their blood pressure readings at home. Although it remains controversial, hypertension may be defined by repeated home BP readings that average ≥ 130/80 mmHg. Ambulatory 24-hour BP monitoring may be a useful adjunct to home or office BP measurements in evaluating patients with marked discrepancies in BP readings, e.g., "*white coat*" (isolated office) hypertension, or "*masked*" (isolated home) hypertension, and in identifying individuals at increased cardiovascular risk, e.g., those without a normal "dip" in BP at night (nocturnal hypertension), or who have a steep surge in BP in the morning or during stress (intermittent hypertension). A diary should be kept as to whether or not stress or problems had occurred on a particular day. It is important to recognize that *BP decreases postprandially* and that this can affect interpretation of the BP reading. Review of the log at the end of several weeks usually identifies the individual who needs treatment, and may help eliminate those who may not require treatment. After starting treatment, the patient should continue to keep a log for you to review. Necessary adjustments in therapy may become evident.

The most important early treatment recommendations should include lifestyle modifications, e.g., weight loss (if overweight), moderation of alcohol consumption, regular physical activity, reduction in sodium intake, and smoking cessation (to reduce cardiovascular risk, not necessarily BP), along with a diet rich in fruits and vegetables (high potassium), and low-fat dairy products (high calcium), with a reduced content of saturated and total fats (DASH diet). (**Figure 18-2**)

Practitioners may differ as to when to start antihypertensive therapy in a patient having milder degrees of blood pressure elevation. Previous practice guidelines set the threshold for beginning pharmacologic treatment at a BP ≥ 140/90 mmHg in most patients with hypertension, and a BP ≥ 150/90 mmHg in older hypertensive adults. However, based on recent clinical trial data, updated guidelines now recommend initiation of antihypertensive therapy at a BP ≥ 140/90 mmHg in all hypertensive patients, and a BP ≥ 130/80 mmHg in individuals at higher risk, i.e., those with known cardiovascular disease, diabetes, chronic kidney disease, or a 10 year ASCVD risk of ≥ 10% (see below). The magnitude of BP elevation should be used to guide the number of antihypertensive agents to start with when implementing drug therapy. For patients with moderate to severe hypertension, more intensive pharmacologic therapy may be warranted, especially if target organ damage is present. Keep in mind that lifestyle modification may be all that is necessary in patients with milder degrees of elevated BP. For example, what is often not recognized is that obese patients may have a return to a normal blood pressure reading once the excess weight is lost. Remember that spurious high blood pressure readings can be recorded in obese individuals if the wrong cuff-size is used. If a larger (more appropriate) size cuff is used, it may reveal a normal blood pressure. Several blood pressure recordings should be recorded on each patient in a given visit. It is not unusual for a drop of 10 to 15 mm Hg in systolic pressure and 5 to 10 mm Hg in diastolic pressure to occur over a period

Figure 18-2

HYPERTENSION TREATMENT ALGORITHM

Aim for target BP goal*
↓

Lifestyle Modifications:

Weight reduction
Moderation of alcohol intake
Regular physical activity
Reduction of sodium intake
Smoking cessation

↓

Not at BP goal
↓

Continue Lifestyle Modifications
Initial Pharmacological Selection:

Try low dose and long acting agent.
In non-black patients, initiate thiazide-type diuretic, ACE inhibitor, ARB, or calcium channel blocker, alone or in combination
In black patients, initiate thiazide-type diuretic or calcium channel blocker, alone or in combination
Low dose combinations may be appropriate (avoid combined use of ACE inhibitor and ARB).

↓

Not at BP goal
↓

| Increase drug dose | Substitute another drug (especially if side effects bothersome) | Add additional agents from a different class (e.g., β-blocker, aldosterone antagonist, or others) |

↓

Not at BP goal
↓

Add a second or third agent.
Most patients will require multiple medications to achieve BP goal.
Inadequate Response**

---

*Note: Previous practice guidelines set the target BP goal at < 140/90 mmHg for most patients with hypertension, and < 150/90 mmHg for older hypertensive adults. However, based on recent clinical trial data, updated guidelines now recommend pharmacologic treatment at a target BP goal of < 140/90 mmHg for all hypertensive patients, and a lower BP goal of < 130/80 mmHg for individuals at higher risk, i.e., those with known cardiovascular disease, diabetes, chronic kidney disease, or a 10 year ASCVD risk of ≥ 10%.
**If not at goal BP, consider referral to a hypertension specialist.

of 5 to 10 minutes. Take the blood pressure in both arms. If a discrepancy exists on the second arm examined, go back to recheck the first arm.

The challenge in the evaluation and treatment of hypertension is identifying the minority (5%) of patients who have potentially curable forms of secondary hypertension and establishing the best BP control regimen for the vast majority of patients with primary hypertension. The extent to which cardiac output, peripheral vascular resistance, intravascular volume, sympathetic nervous system stimulation, and the renin-angiotensin-aldosterone system influence BP differs from patient to patient. Therapy should be individualized as much as possible for each patient. Although essential hypertension has no cure, dietary restriction of sodium and alcohol intake along with lifestyle modifications (including exercise, weight reduction, and stress management) can often control it, especially in early, mild cases. If the BP remains elevated, especially if target organ damage or cardiovascular risk factors are present, the use of one or more of the various antihypertensive drugs currently available may be helpful (**Figure 18-2**).

Ideally, treatment should begin before damage to a vital organ takes place. The vital organs affected by hypertension are the heart, brain, aorta, peripheral vasculature, kidneys, and eyes. Left untreated, ~50% of hypertensive patients die from CAD or CHF, ~33% from stroke, and ~10–15% from complications of renal failure. There are several major categories of drugs available to control hypertension. Keep in mind that the blood pressure (BP) is the product of the cardiac output (CO) and the peripheral vascular resistance (PVR) (BP = CO × PVR). Since the key factors that regulate BP are cardiac output (stroke volume × heart rate) and the peripheral vascular resistance (particularly as mediated through blood vessel constriction), all anti-hypertensive drugs act by reducing either the CO and/or the PVR.

BP can be reduced by:

1. *Diuretics*, which decrease volume overload, particularly thiazide diuretics, e.g., hydrochlorothiazide (HydroDIURIL) and potassium-sparing agents (plus thiazide), e.g., spironolactone (Aldactazide), Dyrenium (Dyazide, Maxzide), amiloride (Moduretic). Loop diuretics, e.g., furosemide (Lasix), bumetanide (Bumex), torsemide (Demadex) are effective in patients with renal insufficiency (serum creatinine >2 mg/dL) and in those with CHF.

2. *Beta blockers*, which block adrenergic receptors in the heart (reduces heart rate and work load), e.g., propranolol (Inderal), metoprolol (Lopressor, Toprol-XL), atenolol (Tenormin), nadolol (Corgard), acebutolol (Sectral), esmolol (Brevibloc).

3. *Centrally acting anti-adrenergic agents*, which reduce sympathetic (adrenergic) outflow from the brain (activates inhibitory α-2 receptors), e.g., clonidine (Catapres), methyldopa (Aldomet). Side effects include drowsiness, dry mouth, fatigue, and orthostatic hypotension. Clonidine is available as a transdermal patch that makes once-a-week dosing possible.

106

Dilating blood vessels with:

4. *α-blockers* (blocks α_1 mediated vasoconstrictors), e.g., terazosin (Hytrin), prazosin (Minipress), doxazosin (Cardura)—not a first choice agent (may induce significant postural hypotension; therefore, first dose should be taken at bedtime).

5. *Alpha-beta-blockers*, e.g., labetalol (Normodyne), (Trandate), carvedilol (Coreg).

6. *ACE inhibitors* (suppresses the synthesis of angiotensin II, a potent vasoconstrictor), e.g., captopril (Capoten), enalapril (Vasotec), lisinopril (Zestril, Prinivil), ramipril (Altace), fosinopril (Monopril), quinapril (Accupril).

7. *ARBs* (antagonizes the angiotensin II receptor of vascular muscle), e.g., losartan (Cozaar), irbesartan (Avapro), candesartan (Atacand), valsartan (Diovan), telmisartan (Micardis), eprosartan (Teveten), especially if intolerant to side-effects of ACE inhibitors (e.g., cough, angioneurotic edema).

8. *Calcium channel blockers* (blocks calcium entry into smooth muscle cells of arterial walls, thereby preventing contraction). These include the dihydropyridines, e.g., nifedipine (Procardia, Adalat), amlodipine (Norvasc), felodipine (Plendil), isradipine (DynaCirc), nisoldipine (Sular), nicardipine (Cardene), clevidipine (Cleviprex), and the non-dihydropyridines, e.g., verapamil (Isoptin, Calan, Verelan), and diltiazem (Cardizem, Tiazac, Dilacor).

9. *Direct renin inhibitors* (blocks the action of renin which decreases the production of angiotensin and promotes vasodilation), e.g., aliskiren (Tekturna).

10. *Direct vasodilators* (relaxes smooth muscle cells which surround blood vessels), e.g., hydralazine (Apresoline), minoxidil (Loniten). Hydralazine may cause a lupus-like syndrome; minoxidil may cause unwanted hair growth. Reflex tachycardia (palpitations) and fluid retention (edema) are also common. These agents can worsen angina in patients with CAD.

In the uncomplicated patient, thiazide-type diuretics, ACE inhibitors, ARBs, or calcium channel blockers, alone or in combination, should be considered as initial therapy for most. Additional drug choices (e.g., β-blockers, aldosterone antagonists, or others) may be used based on the response to the initial therapy and/or as dictated by concomitant medical conditions and the drug's safety, tolerability, cost, and other lifestyle issues (**Figure 18-2** and **18-3**). In certain clinical conditions, there may be compelling indications for specific agents as the initial treatment. For example:

- ACE inhibitors and ARBs in patients with Type I and Type II diabetes with proteinuria (these agents slow the progression of nephropathy in patients with diabetes mellitus)

Figure 18-3

TAILORED PHARMACOLOGIC THERAPY FOR HYPERTENSION

INDICATION	DRUG THERAPY
Types I and II diabetes mellitus with proteinuria	ACE inhibitor Angiotensin II receptor blocker (ARB)
Heart failure	ACE inhibitor Diuretic Beta blocker Angiotensin II receptor blocker (ARB) Aldosterone antagonist
Isolated systolic hypertension (older patient)	Diuretic (preferred) Long-acting dihydropyridine calcium channel blocker
Myocardial infarction	Beta blocker ACE inhibitor or ARB (with systolic dysfunction)
Angina pectoris	Beta blocker Calcium channel blocker (long-acting)
Atrial tachycardia and fibrillation	Beta blocker Non-dihydropyridine calcium channel blocker
Benign prostatic hyperplasia	α -blocker
Essential tremor	Beta blocker (noncardioselective)
Hyperthyroidism	Beta blocker
Migraine	Beta blocker (noncardioselective)
Renal insufficiency	ACE inhibitor Diuretic Calcium channel blocker (non-dihydropyridine)

- Hypertension in African-Americans tends to respond better to diuretics or calcium channel blockers than to beta blockers or ACE inhibitors.
- CHF due to systolic LV dysfunction (ACE inhibitors, diuretics [including spironolactone], beta blockers, e.g., carvedilol [Coreg] as tolerated, and ARBs)
- CHF due to diastolic dysfunction (beta blockers, diuretics, and calcium channel blockers)
- CAD (beta blockers and long-acting calcium channel blockers)

- Isolated systolic hypertension in the elderly (diuretics and long-acting dihydropyridine calcium channel blockers)
- Benign prostatic hypertrophy (alpha blockers, e.g., doxazosin [Cardura], terazosin [Hytrin])
- Aortic regurgitation (ACE inhibitors and nifedipine)
- Migraine headaches (beta blockers and calcium channel blockers [especially verapamil])

While younger patients and those with specific comorbidities (e.g., CAD, CHF, tachyarrhythmias) may exhibit net benefit from using beta blockers as antihypertensive agents, older patients with primary hypertension appear to accrue less benefit and can potentially have an increased risk for stroke.

It is important to consider the patient's lifestyle when prescribing antihypertensive therapy. The adverse physical, mental and metabolic side effects of hypertensive therapy (e.g., fatigue, depression, and erectile dysfunction from beta blockers) may result in nonadherence to prescribed regimens.

The majority of patients with primary hypertension will require 2 or more medications to achieve target BP goal. Most of these regimens include a thiazide-type diuretic (unless absolutely contraindicated). A minority of patients require 3 or more medications in combination. Patients who are compliant with their regimen and who do not respond should be evaluated for secondary causes.

Hypertensive Crises: Emergencies/Urgencies and Other Considerations

An occasional patient with primary or secondary hypertension may enter an accelerated phase characterized by severe arterial hypertension and papilledema, a condition previously known as *malignant hypertension*. Many of these patients also have headache, vomiting, visual disturbances, paralyses, seizures, stupor, or even coma (*hypertensive encephalopathy*). These conditions are now termed *hypertensive emergencies*. The patient with a hypertensive emergency may also present with severe hypertension complicated by evidence of acute target organ dysfunction, e.g., unstable angina, acute MI, pulmonary edema, aortic dissection, preeclampsia-eclampsia, or rapidly deteriorating renal function. Although the actual BP level may not be as important as the rate of BP rise, most end-organ damage is noted with systolic BP > 180 mmHg and/or diastolic BP > 120 mmHg. Management of hypertensive emergencies is often performed in the hospital and by means of intravenous drugs, to reduce the BP as rapidly and safely as possible. The mean arterial BP should be reduced by no more than 25% initially, and then, if the patient is stable, to a BP goal of 160/100-110 mmHg over the next several hours. Larger reductions in BP may worsen target organ dysfunction, particularly in the brain. An exception to this rule is aortic dissection which demands that the BP be reduced quickly to a lower target goal (systolic BP <100-120 mmHg) if tolerated. A growing number of agents are available for management of acute hypertensive syndromes. The appropriate therapeutic approach varies according to the clinical presentation (**Figure 18-4**):

- Drugs available for treatment of hypertensive emergencies include parenteral antihypertensives e.g., nitroprusside (Nipride); nitroglycerin; labetalol (Normodyne, Trandate)—combination beta and alpha blocking effects; esmolol (Brevibloc); enalaprilat (Vasotec); fenoldopam (Corlopam); nicardipine (Cardene); clevidipine (Cleviprex); and phentolamine (Regitine).
- Nitroprusside in combination with a beta blocker is especially useful in patients with aortic dissection. Thiocyanate levels should be monitored when using nitroprusside, since cyanide toxicity may occur with high doses, prolonged infusion, or when hepatic or renal impairment is present.
- With myocardial ischemia, IV nitroglycerin or an intravenous beta blocker, e.g., labetalol or esmolol, is preferable.
- ACE inhibitors (and ARBs) slow the progression of nephropathy in patients with diabetes mellitus, and are first line agents in this setting. The practitioner should keep in mind that the dosage of ACE inhibitors needs to be reduced in the presence of renal failure and that these agents (along with ARBs) are contraindicated in pregnancy because they may cause adverse effects on the fetus.
- Methyldopa is the drug of choice in pregnancy because of its proven safety. Hydralazine, labetalol, and calcium channel blockers are also safe and can be used as alternative agents.

Figure 18-4

TREATMENT OF HYPERTENSIVE EMERGENCIES

- **Myocardial ischemia**
  —Nitroglycerin, and beta-blockers
- **Pulmonary edema**
  —Loop diuretic, nitroprusside, nitroglycerin
- **Aortic dissection**
  —Type A–surgery
  —Type B–labetalol, or nitroprusside with a beta blocker (Avoid medications that predispose to reflex tachycardia)
- **Hypertensive encephalopathy**
  —Sodium nitroprusside, or labetalol
- **Pheochromocytoma (a catecholamine-secreting tumor)**
  —Phentolamine (an alpha blocker)

Patients with less severe hypertensive syndromes, i.e., *hypertensive urgencies*, have no evidence of acute target organ dysfunction and can often be treated with oral therapy. When the BP has been brought under control, combinations of oral antihypertensive agents can be substituted as parenteral drugs are tapered off.

Antihypertensive medication must be used with caution in certain settings. For example:

- Beta blockers may induce bronchospasm in patients with lung disease.

- ACE inhibitors may worsen renal function, especially with renal artery stenosis (In renal artery stenosis, the kidney needs a high efferent glomerular arteriolar resistance for successful filtration; ACE inhibitors reduce the arteriolar resistance and may result in renal failure).

- Thiazide diuretics are ineffective when the serum creatinine is >2.5 mg/dL.

- Spironolactone may induce hyperkalemia when combined with ACE inhibitors/ARBs or if marked renal insufficiency is present.

- Alpha blockers may induce postural hypotension and should be used with caution in the elderly.

- ACE inhibitors, ARBs, and direct renin inhibitors should be avoided in pregnancy.

- Abruptly stopping clonidine may lead to rebound hypertension.

- Beta blockers may precipitate a hypertensive crisis in patients with pheochromocytoma if given alone or before alpha blockers by leaving α-adrenergic stimulation unopposed.

- The combination of obesity, hypertension, hyperglycemia (adult onset [type II] diabetes mellitus), elevated triglycerides and low HDL cholesterol levels are clues to the *metabolic or insulin resistance syndrome*. Thiazide diuretics should be used with caution since they may exacerbate insulin resistance, and as a result, raise serum glucose levels. Keep in mind that beta blockers may raise triglyceride levels, lower HDL cholesterol levels, promote weight gain, and increase the incidence of new onset diabetes (compared with other antihypertensive drugs).

Hypertension therapy should start with a low dose of a long-acting once-daily drug (preferably a thiazide-type diuretic) and titrate the dose to manage side effects and maximize compliance. If no response, or bothersome side effects occur, another drug from another class should be substituted. If the response is inadequate, but the drug is well tolerated, a second agent from a different class should be added. Although updated BP goals for older hypertensive patients are the same as for younger patients, it is advisable to "start low and go slow".

- Drugs that may exaggerate postural hypotension or cause cognitive dysfunction should be used with caution.

- The peripheral vasodilator SL nifedipine (Procardia) should be avoided due to its unpredictable, and often dramatic and precipitous decrease in

BP, along with the reflex increase in heart rate and its attendant threat of damage to the brain or myocardium from hypoperfusion. Elderly patients and those with volume depletion are at particular risk of hypotension during treatment.

Blood Pressure Goal and Choice of Drug Therapy

Considerable controversy surrounds the optimal BP goal for the treatment of hypertension. Previous practice guidelines set the BP goal for most adults with hypertension at <140/90 mmHg, irrespective of age, and <130/80 mmHg (based largely on expert opinion) for those with diabetes or chronic kidney disease. Observational studies demonstrated that lower BP is better than higher, and many trials have confirmed that treatment of hypertension is beneficial. Over the years, however, clinical trial data called into question the concept of "lower is better", and failed to show evidence of significant clinical benefit of "intensive" over "standard" BP control in reducing cardiovascular event rates (with the exception of a small reduction in the risk of stroke), and suggested the potential for harm with overly aggressive therapy (so-called "J curve" phenomenon). Accordingly, an expert panel of the eighth Joint National Committee (JNC 8) on the management of hypertension in adults issued updated "evidence – based" guidelines that recommended a less stringent BP goal of <140/90 mmHg for patients with diabetes or chronic kidney disease, the same as for the general population of adults under the age of 60. A slightly more relaxed (and controversial) BP goal of < 150/90 mmHg was recommended for patients age 60 or older, based on prior evidence showing little additional benefit from achieving a lower BP target. However, not all experts agreed with the revised BP goal for patients over the age of 60, arguing that the evidence does not support the change, and that a less aggressive BP goal may lead to harmful consequences. Other U.S. and international practice guidelines set similar, less intensive BP goals of <140/90 mmHg for "high risk" patients (i.e., those with diabetes, chronic kidney disease or ASCVD) and < 150/90 mmHg for older hypertensive adults, however, the age cutoff (80 years as opposed to 60 years) is higher in some than in the JNC 8 guidelines, and according to many experts, better reflects when treatment-related adverse events, e.g., dizziness and falls, are more likely to occur. Caution is advised against lowering diastolic BP to below 60 mmHg, particularly in CAD patients over the age of 60, since it may reduce coronary perfusion and worsen myocardial ischemia.

Adding more fuel to the debate are the results of a recent "landmark" clinical trial that has shown a beneficial effect of an aggressive systolic BP goal of < 120 mmHg as compared to <140 mmHg in reducing cardiovascular event rates (CHF, but not MI or stroke) and mortality, albeit at a cost of additional medication side effects, e.g., hypotension, syncope, and acute kidney injury, in "high risk" non-diabetic hypertensive adults age 50 years and older. Of note, BP measurements in this trial were taken unattended (to minimize "white-coat" effect) using an automated device, which tend to be 5-10 mmHg lower than if taken manually (auscultatory method). As a result, updated guidelines now recommend a more intensive manual (auscultatory) BP target of <130/80 mmHg in patients with, or at high risk for, cardiovascular disease, if it can be achieved without producing significant medication side effects. Regardless of the BP goal, BP reduction should be gradual and treatment individualized ("one size does not fit all"), and should be accompanied by appropriate lifestyle modifications and management of other cardiovascular risk factors.

As primary preventive therapy, β-blockers are less effective than other antihypertensive agents at reducing the risk of stroke, lack cardiovascular morbidity and mortality benefit, and have adverse metabolic effects. Therefore, for non-black patients with uncomplicated hypertension without known CAD, preference should be given to ACE inhibitors, ARBs, calcium channel blockers, and thiazide-type diuretics. For black patients, initial therapy should include a thiazide-type diuretic or calcium channel blocker. For patients with chronic kidney disease, initial (or add-on) therapy should include an ACE inhibitor or ARB (not both combined), to preserve renal function, with close monitoring of potassium and serum creatinine levels. The combination of an ACE inhibitor plus a calcium channel blocker has recently been shown to be effective initial therapy, possibly superior to the combination of an ACE inhibitor (or a β-blocker) and a thiazide diuretic. However, chlorthalidone is longer acting than hydrochlorothiazide, provides greater 24 hour BP reduction, and may be associated with better clinical outcomes. For the management of hypertension in patients with established CAD (stable or unstable angina, non ST or ST elevation MI), β-blockers along with ACE inhibitors or ARBs are the treatment of choice. If further BP lowering is needed, a thiazide diuretic and/or a dihydropyridine calcium channel blocker, e.g., amlodipine, can be added. If a β-blocker is contraindicated or not tolerated, a non-dihydropyridine calcium channel blocker, e.g., diltiazem or verapamil, can be substituted. If there is LV systolic dysfunction, recommended therapy consists of an ACE inhibitor or ARB, a β-blocker, and either a thiazide or loop diuretic. In patients with more severe heart failure, an aldosterone antagonist and direct-acting vasodilators, e.g., hydralazine/isosorbide dinitrate (in African American patients) should be considered.

Resistant Hypertension

Resistant hypertension is defined as a BP that remains elevated despite the use of 3 or more antihypertensive medications (including a diuretic) at optimal dosages. Successful treatment of patients with resistant hypertension requires consideration of lifestyle factors that contribute to treatment resistance, e.g., obesity, dietary salt intake, and alcohol consumption; diagnosing and treating secondary causes of hypertension, e.g., drug-related causes (NSAIDs, steroids, oral contraceptives, decongestants, diet pills, cocaine, licorice, amphetamine-like stimulants, ephedra, cyclosporine, and erythropoietin), obstructive sleep apnea, chronic kidney disease, primary aldosteronism, and renal artery stenosis; and using multiple drug treatments with different mechanisms of action effectively. In this regard, a generally useful strategy for most patients with resistant hypertension is to combine an ACE inhibitor or ARB, together with a long acting calcium channel blocker (e.g., amlodipine), and a thiazide-like diuretic (preferably chlorthalidone). If the BP remains uncontrolled despite an optimized 3-drug regimen, other antihypertensive medications e.g., an aldosterone antagonist (spironolactone, eplerenone), vasodilating β-blocker (combined α-/ β-blocker [e.g., carvedilol, labetalol] or nebivolol), pure α-blocker (e.g., terazosin, doxazosin), central acting antiadrenergic agent (e.g., clonidine), and direct vasodilator (e.g., hydralazine, minoxidil) can be added as needed. Among specific classes of antihypertensive medications, diuretics are the most useful (and most underused) agents in the management of resistant hypertension. Medications that antagonize mineralocorticoid receptor actions i.e., aldosterone antagonists, e.g., spironolactone, can further reduce BP among patients receiving multiple antihypertensive medications, particularly those with primary aldosteronism (which is found in ~20% of patients with resistant hypertension). Loop diuretics should be considered in patients with chronic kidney disease and/or those receiving potent vasodilators (e.g., minoxidil).

Evaluation of patients with resistant hypertension should be directed at confirming true treatment resistance. Excluding "pseudo-resistance" due to poor patient adherence to therapy (one of the leading causes of uncontrolled hypertension) or a "white-coat" effect may require more frequent office visits and home, work, or 24 hour ambulatory BP monitoring. The central acting alpha-2 agonist clonidine is a poor choice in intermittently compliant patients due to sudden rebound hypertension that may result if the drug is abruptly stopped. Since complex dosing regimens are associated with poor patient compliance, prescribed regimens should be simplified as much as possible. Dosing some antihypertensive medications at night may reduce BP to a greater degree than dosing during the day. If the BP remains uncontrolled after 6 months of treatment or a specific secondary cause of hypertension is suspected, referral to an appropriate specialist is recommended.

It should be noted, however, that despite focused efforts on lifestyle modification and aggressive pharmacological treatment strategies, a significant number of patients with resistant hypertension fail to achieve adequate BP control, even under expert-guided care, and remain at high risk for a major cardiovascular event. (**Note:** Cardiovascular risk doubles with each increment of 20/10 mmHg in BP). Evidence suggests that treatment failure in these patients may be due, at least in part, to over-activation of the sympathetic nervous system. Recently developed interventional therapies targeting excess sympathetic neural activity, either directly by radiofrequency catheter ablation of the renal artery sympathetic nerves (*renal sympathetic denervation*), or indirectly by electrical activation of the carotid baroreflex via a surgically implantable pacemaker-like baroreceptor stimulation device (*carotid baroreflex activation*), are currently undergoing active investigation. Although results from preliminary clinical trials have been promising, subsequent clinical trial data has failed to show a significant benefit of renal sympathetic denervation in lowering BP when compared to a placebo. However, the results from more recent studies suggest benefit. As a result, the future role of these novel device-based therapies in the management of treatment-resistant hypertension is uncertain.

Chapter 19.   Dyslipidemia

Atherosclerotic cardiovascular disease (ASCVD) is the leading cause of morbidity and mortality in the United States. Dyslipidemia, i.e., elevated serum levels of total and LDL cholesterol, low HDL cholesterol, and/or high triglycerides, is a powerful risk factor for atherosclerosis, and its proper identification and treatment, particularly LDL cholesterol reduction with a statin, the cornerstone in the primary and secondary prevention of CAD. This chapter will provide an overview of plasma lipids, their role in the pathogenesis of atherosclerosis, and the practical approach to the patient who presents with dyslipidemia.

Lipids and Atherosclerosis

Lipids, e.g., cholesterol and triglycerides, are transported around the body by particles called lipoproteins. These lipoproteins contain surface proteins, known as apoproteins (apo), that help guide lipid transport and metabolism. Lipoproteins can be classified as high density lipoprotein (HDL), intermediate density lipoprotein (IDL), low density lipoprotein (LDL), very low density lipoprotein (VLDL), and chylomicrons. All lipoprotein fractions play a role in atherogenesis. Two major apo B containing lipoproteins, cholesterol-rich LDL (especially small, dense LDL) and its genetic variant, lipoprotein (a), and triglyceride-rich VLDL, promote atherosclerosis, whereas apo A-1 containing HDL cholesterol inhibits the process due to HDL's ability to transport lipids away from the vessel walls back to the liver for disposal (so-called "reverse cholesterol transport"). The development of atherosclerosis is a complex interaction between genetic predisposition, CAD risk factors, endothelial dysfunction, lipid accumulation (mainly oxidized LDL), vascular inflammation, and arterial thrombosis. Dyslipidemia has emerged as a major modifiable risk factor and clinical trials have clearly demonstrated the benefits of pharmacologic lipid reduction, especially LDL cholesterol lowering with a statin, in patients with or at risk for CAD. The lipid "hypothesis", therefore, is no longer a theory, it is a fact! Numerous primary and secondary prevention studies have demonstrated a nearly 30% reduction rate in CAD death or non-fatal MI with statin therapy.

The most important prognostic feature of CAD is the stability or instability of the coronary atherosclerotic plaque. A previously unstable (but nonobstructive and noncalcified) lipid-rich and inflammatory plaque can rupture with sudden partial or total occlusion from coronary thrombosis, resulting in an acute coronary syndrome (unstable angina, acute MI) or sudden cardiac death. These unstable plaques that are vulnerable to rupture are usually not large and appear on coronary angiography to obstruct <70% of the arterial lumen. This explains why a patient may have no symptoms, a normal resting ECG, exercise stress test, and cardiovascular examination, and even a negative electron beam computerized tomography (EBCT) scan, and have a heart attack soon thereafter! The stability or instability of a coronary plaque is not discernible by EBCT or routine coronary angiography. Elevated serum LDL-cholesterol levels, however, are a major contributor to the development of the unstable coronary plaque. HMG-coenzyme A reductase inhibitors ("statins"), for example, can lower LDL cholesterol, decrease lipid deposition in the arterial wall, reduce inflammation (as measured by reduction in C-reactive protein), improve endothelial dysfunction, stabilize the plaque and make it less likely to rupture. (**Note:** A 1% reduction in LDL cholesterol level correlates with ~1% reduction in CAD rates.) Aggressive lipid-lowering therapy with a statin should be strongly encouraged in both the primary (patients without evident CAD) and secondary (patients with known vascular disease) prevention of CAD. Beta blockers and ACE inhibitors can also stabilize plaques. A ruptured plaque may heal or result in clot formation, often with more severe stenosis. Keep in mind that aspirin helps to prevent clot formation and is effective in reducing primary and secondary coronary events.

Therapeutic Considerations

Dyslipidemia is usually asymptomatic, but may on rare occasion be discovered when physical signs of hyperlipidemia (e.g., xanthelasmas, corneal arcus, xanthomas) or more commonly when abnormal lipid levels are detected during routine examination or evaluation of a patient. Therapeutic lifestyle changes, e.g., diet and exercise, are mainstays of lipid management. Lifestyle changes alone, however, rarely reduce LDL cholesterol more than 10–20%. As an adjunct to lifestyle interventions, there are seven major classes of drugs that are used to treat lipid disorders (**Figure 19-1**). Before starting lipid therapy, however, a potentially reversible secondary cause of dyslipidemia, e.g., hypothyroidism, poorly controlled diabetes, obesity, excess alcohol use, or drugs (e.g., thiazide diuretics, β-Blockers, estrogens, steroids, protease inhibitors) should be searched for and corrected if possible. In general, the higher the overall CAD risk, the lower should be the LDL-cholesterol.

According to previous practice guidelines, risk factors that modify treatment goals for LDL cholesterol include:

- Cigarette smoking
- Hypertension
- Low HDL (< 40 mg/dL); High HDL (≥ 60mg/dL) is a "negative" risk (subtract 1 risk factor)
- Positive family history of coronary artery disease (Men, first degree relative < 55 years) (Women, first degree relative < 65 years)
- Age (Men ≥ 45 years)(Women ≥ 55 years)

Figure 19-1

TREATMENT OF DYSLIPIDEMIA

DRUG	LDL	HDL	TG	SIDE EFFECTS
HMG-CoA reductase inhibitors (Statins) **Lovastatin (Mevacor)** **Pravastatin (Pravachol)**	↓ 18–55%	↑ 5–15%	↓ 7–30%	Hepatotoxicity⎫ dose- Myopathy ⎬ dependent ⎭ (especially high dose simvastatin)*
Simvastatin (Zocor) Atorvastatin (Lipitor) Fluvastatin (Lescol) Rosuvastatin (Crestor) Pitavastatin (Livalo)				Small ↑ risk of new onset diabetes and cognitive dysfunction (outweighed by ↓ CAD events and ↓ mortality) Potential drug interactions
Bile acid sequestrants (Resins) **Cholestyramine (Questran)** **Colestipol (Colestid)** **Colesevelam (Welchol)**	↓ 15–30%	↑ 3–5%	may ↑	GI distress, constipation, bloating
Fibrates **Gemfibrozil (Lopid)** **Fenofibrate (Tricor)** **Fenofibric acid (Trilipix)**	↓ 5–20%	↑ 10–35%	↓ 20–50%	GI distress, nausea, gallstones Myopathy (when with statin)— especially gemfibrozil
Nicotinic acid (Niacin)	↓ 5–25%	↑ 15–35%	↓ 20–50%	Flushing (may be relieved by aspirin), pruritus, GI distress, exacerbates peptic ulcer disease, hyperglycemia, hyperuricemia (or gout), hepatotoxicity
Cholesterol absorption inhibitors **Ezetimibe (Zetia)**	↓ 18–20%	↑ 1–5%	↓ 5–11%	Generally well tolerated. Slightly more fatigue, GI distress, muscle and back pain compared to placebo Hepatotoxicity (when with statin)

Figure 19-1

TREATMENT OF DYSLIPIDEMIA (*Continued*)

DRUG	LDL	HDL	TG	SIDE EFFECTS
Omega-3 fatty acids Fish oil (Lovaza) (Vascepa)	may ↑ (Lovaza only)	↑ 5–10%	↓ 20–50%	GI distress, nausea, fishy after taste, may increase bleeding when used with antiplatelet or anticoagulant agents.
PCSK9 inhibitors Alirocumab (Praluent) Evolocumab (Repatha)	↓ 40-65%	↑ 5–10%	↓ 15–25%	Myalgias, rash, urticaria, cognitive effects, mild injection-site reactions

*Note: Doubling of statin dose lowers LDL cholesterol by 6%, but increases risk of myopathy and hepatitis. Risk of myopathy increases significantly with 80 mg dose of simvastatin (avoid unless dose already tolerated > 12 months).

The cholesterol-lowering agents have long been used to achieve a primary goal target LDL cholesterol level of:

- <160 mg/dL if no CAD and 0–1 risk factors
- <130 mg/dL if no CAD and > 2 risk factors
- <100 mg/dL if CAD, PAD, AAA, carotid artery disease, and/or diabetes mellitus is present. Those with ACS, CAD and multiple risk factors or diabetes are at very high risk and a target LDL cholesterol level of <70 mg/dL has been the goal. For individuals who have a low HDL cholesterol and a high triglyceride level, secondary goals have included a target HDL cholesterol of >40 mg/dL, a triglyceride level of <150 mg/dL, a "non-HDL" cholesterol (total cholesterol – HDL cholesterol) level 30 mg/dL higher than the target LDL cholesterol goals, and an apo B level (a measure of the total number of atherogenic lipoprotein particles) of <90 mg/dL (or <80 mg/dL if at very high risk).

CAD is preventable. In concert with reduction of other CAD risk factors (e.g., cigarette smoking, hypertension, diabetes mellitus), all patients over age 20 should be screened for elevated total and LDL-cholesterol, reduced HDL-cholesterol, and elevated triglycerides at least once every 5 years. Keep in mind that when you order a lipid profile, the usual lipids measured directly are total cholesterol, HDL cholesterol and triglycerides. In general, the higher the HDL (so-called "good") cholesterol (which protects the arteries against the build-up of fatty deposits) and the lower the triglycerides, the better. The level of LDL cholesterol (referred to as "bad" cholesterol since it causes fatty deposits to build up in the arteries) is a valuable clue to determining the risk for ASCVD. Another lipoprotein, Lp(a), is associated with increased risk for CAD, but treatment with statins does not lower Lp(a) levels or risk. Small LDL particles and HDL subfractions are related to CAD, but are not superior to LDL or HDL in predicting risk. Measurement of these other lipoproteins is not routinely indicated.

Although LDL cholesterol can be measured directly, it is more commonly calculated indirectly by clinical laboratories using the following formula: *LDL cholesterol* = total cholesterol − HDL cholesterol − (*triglyceride/5*). (**Note:** If the triglyceride level is >400 mg/dL, this formula will not be accurate.) Total cholesterol and HDL cholesterol levels can be measured at any time of the day in the non-fasting state, but triglyceride levels should be measured only from fasting patients (at least 12–14 hours after eating) because triglycerides increase after a fatty meal. It is important to keep this in mind since *the higher the triglycerides, the lower the calculated LDL cholesterol*. Thus, LDL cholesterol may be falsely low in the non-fasting state, rather than elevated (as is sometimes assumed). Cholesterol levels measured within the first 24 hours post-MI reflect pre-event lipid values. Cholesterol values fall markedly (and triglyceride levels rise), however, in the week post-MI and remain low for up to 1 month. Patients who recently had a MI, therefore, should be tested at a later time. Lipid determinations are best carried out in stable ambulatory patients.

Previous practice guidelines focused primarily on reducing LDL cholesterol by at least 30–40%, particularly with a statin. The exception is the case of very high triglycerides (>500–1000 mg/dL) which requires urgent correction to prevent acute pancreatitis. If adequate LDL cholesterol lowering can not be achieved with statin therapy alone, either ezetimibe, a bile acid sequestrant, or niacin may be added; however, proof of clinical benefit for the latter two is lacking. In patients with triglyceride levels >200 mg/dL, non-HDL cholesterol (a surrogate marker of apo B) has been the next target, and the clinician may consider adding a fibrate or niacin to statin therapy. Although low HDL cholesterol is associated with an increased risk for CAD, there is no clearcut evidence of cardiovascular benefit from treating this disorder. Since elevated triglycerides are often associated with other lipid abnormalities, e.g., low HDL cholesterol levels and small dense LDL particles (atherogenic dyslipidemia), along with a cluster of other risk factors (e.g., abdominal obesity, hypertension, and fasting hyperglycemia) as part of the *metabolic syndrome*, treatment of high risk patients with niacin, a fibrate, or fish oil in addition to statin therapy seems reasonable. (**Figure 19-2**) Both fibrates and niacin lower triglycerides, raise HDL cholesterol, and can shift small, dense ("pattern B") LDL particles that are highly atherogenic to larger, more buoyant and fluffy ("pattern A") LDL particles which are less atherogenic. Refractory cases of hypertriglyceridemia may benefit from omega-3 fatty acids (fish oil supplements) which, by reducing VLDL production, can lower the triglyceride level by 20–50%. If multiple drug therapy is being considered, lipid levels, along with liver enzymes, e.g., transaminases and creatinine kinase (clues to hepatotoxicity and myopathy, respectively) should be monitored as needed.

Figure 19-2

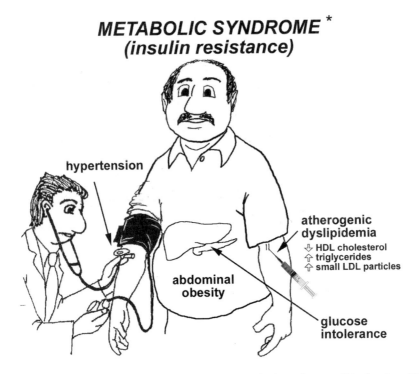

METABOLIC SYNDROME *
(insulin resistance)

hypertension

atherogenic
dyslipidemia
⇩ HDL cholesterol
⇧ triglycerides
⇧ small LDL particles

abdominal
obesity

glucose
intolerance

*Note: Metabolic syndrome includes ≥3 of the following: waist circumference >40 in. (men) or >35 in. (women); triglycerides >150 mg/dL; HDL cholesterol <40 mg/dL (men) or <50 mg/dL (women); BP >130/85 mmHg; fasting glucose >100 mg/dL.

It should be realized, however, that the target lipid levels that have long been recommended by practice guidelines have not been based on solid clinical trial evidence. Furthermore, despite improvements in the lipid profile, no oral cholesterol lowering drugs with the exception of ezetimibe, have been shown to offer significant cardiovascular benefit over statin therapy alone. Accordingly, the American Heart Association issued updated "evidence-based" guidelines on cholesterol management that shifted the focus away from treatment to specific LDL (and non-HDL) cholesterol targets to reduction in overall cardiovascular risk with therapeutic lifestyle changes, along with the use of moderate to high intensity statin therapy which, by virtue of its LDL cholesterol lowering (by at least 30-50%) and pleiotropic (e.g., antiinflammatory, antithrombotic) effects, has been shown to be beneficial in the primary and secondary prevention of atherosclerotic cardiovascular disease (ASCVD). Four groups of patients who derive the most benefit from statin therapy, regardless of the baseline lipid levels, have been identified. These include patients who already have ASCVD (CAD, stroke/TIA, peripheral artery disease [PAD]); those with an LDL-cholesterol of ≥ 190 mg/dL (i.e., familial hypercholesterolemia); individuals aged 40 to 75 years with diabetes; and those who have an estimated 10 year risk of ASCVD of at least 7.5%, based on a new risk calculator (which some experts claim may overestimate risk) that factors in age, gender, race, cholesterol levels, BP, diabetes and smoking status. If risk remains unclear, other factors, e.g., family history of premature ASCVD, high sensitivity C-reactive protein (a marker of inflammation), coronary calcium score, and ankle brachial index may be considered (**Figure 19-3**). Due to the lack of clinical trial evidence, nonstatin therapies, alone or in combination with a statin, are not recommended as first line treatment to reduce ASCVD risk. However, non-statin lipid controlling agents e.g., ezetimibe, may

Figure 19-3

TREATMENT OF BLOOD CHOLESTEROL TO REDUCE ATHERO- SCLEROTIC CARDIOVASCULAR RISK IN ADULTS

PATIENT GROUPS		TREATMENT
With atherosclerotic cardiovascular disease and ≥ 21 years of age	≤ 75 years of age	High intensity statin
	> 75 years of age	Moderate intensity statin
With an LDL cholesterol level of ≥ 190 mg/dL	–	High intensity statin
With a 10 year ASCVD risk of ≥ 7.5%	–	High intensity statin
With type 1 or 2 diabetes and ages 40-75 years	–	Moderate intensity statin
With a 10 year ASCVD risk of ≥ 7.5% and ages 40–75 years	–	Moderate to high intensity statin

Note: High intensity statin lowers LDL cholesterol by ≥50%; moderate intensity statin lowers LDL cholesterol by 30-50%.

Adapted from Stone, NJ, Robinson J, Lichtenstein AH, et al. AHA/ACC guidelines on the treatment of blood cholesterol to reduce atherosclerotic cardiovascular risk in adults. J Am Coll Cardiol, 2013.

be considered in patients who have an inadequate response to statin therapy or are statin-intolerant since more recent clinical trial data has shown that the addition of ezetimibe to a statin in high risk ACS patients provides incremental cardiovascular benefit over statin therapy alone. Novel cholesterol lowering therapies, e.g., injectable (subcutaneous) monoclonal antibodies (alirocumab [Praluent], evolocumab [Repatha]) that inhibit the function of proprotein convertase subtilisin-kexin type 9, so-called *PCSK9 inhibitors*, lower LDL cholesterol substantially more than ezetimibe (by 40–70%). These agents have recently been approved as an adjunct to statin therapy for high risk patients with heterozygous familial hypercholesterolemia or known ASCVD, and hold promise as alternative therapy for patients who are statin-intolerant. Results from preliminary clinical trials have been encouraging. Long term cardiovascular outcome data will help establish the role of these powerful (and more costly) new cholesterol lowering agents in ASCVD risk management.

Pearls:

- In addition to therapeutic lifestyle changes, statins (by virtue of their LDL cholesterol lowering and pleiotropic effects) are the drugs of choice for primary and secondary prevention of ASCVD.

- Four groups of patients who derive the most benefit from statin therapy include those with ASCVD, an LDL cholesterol ≥190 mg/dL, diabetes mellitus (ages 40–75 years), and an estimated 10 year ASCVD risk ≥7.5%.

- When considering the "cluster" of risk factors in the patient with metabolic syndrome, keep in mind the mnemonic "**HOLD**" (**H**ypertension, **O**besity, **L**ipid disorders, **D**iabetes).

- Although low HDL cholesterol is linked to increased ASCVD risk, no lipid controlling therapy has been shown to offer significant cardiovascular benefit from treating this disorder.

- In patients intolerant to high dose statins, lower doses or a different statin may be tried on alternate days (or with coenzyme Q10), before switching to other cholesterol lowering drugs.

- In patients with very high risk ASCVD, it is reasonable to add ezetimibe or a PCSK9 inhibitor to maximally tolerated statin therapy if the LDL cholesterol remains ≥ 70 mg/dL ("lower is better").

- In intermediate risk patients for whom the treatment decision is uncertain, statin therapy may be withheld if the coronary artery calcium score is zero, unless other risk enhancing factors, e.g., cigarette smoking, diabetes, or a strong family history of premature ASCVD are present.

Chapter 20. Cardiac Arrhythmias and Conduction Disturbances

Electrical disturbances of the heart result from abnormal impulse formation and/ or conduction, and may range from a benign, incidental finding, to a potentially life-threatening condition. This chapter will present a practical clinical approach to the pharmacologic management of the patient who presents with a cardiac arrhythmia or conduction abnormality, with an emphasis on the most common rate and rhythm disorders encountered in daily practice.

Figure 20-1 summarizes the approach to the more common tachyarrhythmias.

Atrial Fibrillation

Atrial fibrillation is the most common sustained supraventricular arrhythmia encountered in clinical practice, affecting an estimated 5.2 million Americans. The incidence increases with age, so that the lifetime risk for developing atrial fibrillation is nearly 25% for individuals over age 40. Modifiable risk factors for atrial fibrillation include hypertension, diabetes mellitus, obesity, alcohol consumption ("holiday heart"), and obstructive sleep apnea. Atrial fibrillation occurs with many forms of structural heart disease including mitral valve disease, CAD, dilated cardiomyopathy, CHF, atrial septal defect, as well as in other settings, e.g., hyperthyroidism, pericarditis, COPD (as well as with pulmonary medications, e.g., theophylline and beta-adrenergic agonists), and after cardiac surgery. Many patients with atrial fibrillation have no structural heart disease (i.e., "lone" atrial fibrillation, neurogenic atrial fibrillation). Occasionally it is familial. Atrial fibrillation can be classified into three main types: paroxysmal (lasts less than 7 days), persistent (does not terminate spontaneously but can be pharmacologically or electrically converted to sinus rhythm), or permanent.

Therapy options for atrial fibrillation include:

1. *Control ventricular rate,* even if the fibrillation itself is not corrected, with beta blockers, calcium channel blockers (e.g., verapamil, diltiazem), or digoxin, which reduces symptoms and avoids a tachycardia-induced cardiomyopathy.

2. *Restore and maintain normal sinus rhythm through cardioversion or antiarrhythmic agents.* Cardioversion preserves AV synchrony, maintains cardiac output, reduces symptoms and may decrease risk of future thromboembolism. Cardioversion may be applied:

123

Figure 20-1

CLINICAL APPROACH TO COMMON ARRHYTHMIAS

ARRHYTHMIA	PREDISPOSING CONDITIONS	TREATMENT
Atrial premature contractions (premature impulse originates from ectopic foci in the atria)	Normal individual or due to anxiety, caffeine, alcohol, CHF, hypoxemia, electrolyte abnormality ($\downarrow K^+$, $\downarrow Mg^{++}$)	Remove precipitating cause. Treatment rarely required. If symptomatic—β-blocker.
Sinus tachycardia (rapid impulse formation from the SA node)	Fever, pain, anemia, dehydration, CHF, hyperthyroidism, COPD, autonomic disorder (POTS).	Treat the underlying cause, e.g., pain, fever, anemia, anxiety, hypovolemia, CHF, beta-agonists. If symptomatic—β-blocker.
Supraventricular tachycardia —AV nodal reentrant tachycardia (AVNRT) (reentry using dual pathways in the AV node) —AV reciprocating tachycardia (AVRT) (reentry using accessory pathway)	Normal individual or due to preexcitation (WPW) syndrome.	Acutely–vagal maneuvers (abruptly converts to sinus rhythm or no effect at all). If unsuccessful, adenosine, verapamil, β-blocker. Cardioversion (if hemodynamically unstable). Avoid AV nodal blockers in WPW syndrome (can accelerate conduction via bypass tract and precipitate ventricular fibrillation). RF ablation is useful for preventing recurrence.
Atrial fibrillation (wavelets of activation in the atria irregularly passing down the AV node)	Idiopathic ("lone"), mitral valve disease, hypertension, pericarditis, hyperthyroidism, obstructive sleep apnea, COPD, alcohol, post cardiac surgery.	1. Slow the ventricular rate (β-blocker, verapamil, cardizem, digoxin). 2. Convert to sinus rhythm (after anticoagulation if chronic) with IV Ibutilide, Procainamide, Amiodarone, or orally with group IC, III, or IA agent. May require elective cardioversion (likelihood of success dependent on duration of atrial fibrillation and size of atria).
Atrial flutter (macroreentry within the atria)		3. RF ablation for common type atrial flutter and atrial fibrillation (foci in or near pulmonary veins and posterior LA wall). If not successful, try AV node ablation and permanent pacemaker.

124

Multifocal atrial tachycardia (increased automaticity at multiple sites in the atria)	Severe COPD	Treat underlying lung disease. Verapamil may be used to slow ventricular rate. K^+, Mg^{++} supplement. AV node ablation and permanent pacemaker.
Ventricular premature contractions (premature impulse originates from ectopic foci in the ventricle)	CAD, MI, cardiomyopathy, CHF, hypoxemia, $\downarrow K^+$	May not require therapy. If symptomatic—β-blocker
Ventricular tachycardia (3 or more consecutive PVCs) —Monomorphic and polymorphic —Nonsustained VT: lasts <.30 seconds —Sustained VT: lasts > 30 seconds	CAD, MI, cardiomyopathy CHF, hypoxemia, $\downarrow K^+$, arrhythmogenic RV dysplasia/cardiomyopathy, or idiopathic (i.e., no structural heart disease).	May not require therapy. If symptomatic—β -blocker. If unstable–electrical cardioversion. Acute–IV amiodarone, procainamide, lidocaine. Chronic prevention po Class IA, IB, IC, III drugs. Implantable cardioverter defibrillator in patients at high risk of sudden cardiac death. Idiopathic VT may respond to vagal maneuvers, adenosine, verapamil, and β -blocker (RV outflow tract VT), or verapamil, but not adenosine or β -blocker (LV fascicular VT), RF ablation can be curative.
Torsades de pointes (A type of polymorphic VT in which QRS morphology twists around the baseline)	↑QT interval (congenital or drugs e.g., Class IA and III antiarrhythmics, tricyclic antidepressants, antibiotics (e.g., erythromycin, trimethoprim-sulfa), antihistamines (astemizole, terfenadine), hypokalemia, hypomagnesemia, antipsychotics (e.g., phenothiazines, haloperidol).	In acquired long QT, IV magnesium, overdrive pacing (which shortens QT interval), and IV isoproterenol (unless CAD present) which increases the heart rate. Drugs that ↑QT interval are contraindicated. In congenital long QT, β-blockers if symptomatic. Implantable cardioverter defibrillator if syncope or VT despite β-blocker therapy.

- Urgently in unstable patients (ongoing angina, CHF, hypotension), or
- Electively in stable patients, either electrically or with certain antiarrhythmic agents, e.g., the Class III agents, ibutilide (Corvert), amiodarone (Cordarone, Pacerone), sotalol (Betapace), and dofetilide (Tikosyn); the Class IA agents, e.g., procainamide (Pronestyl, Procan) and disopyramide (Norpace), or the Class IC agents, e.g., flecainide (Tambocor) and propafenone (Rythmol). Cardioversion should be considered in stable patients with atrial fibrillation if the rhythm disturbance has been present for <48 hours, or an LA thrombus has been ruled out (by TEE) or effectively treated (international normalized ratio [INR] of 2–3) with warfarin (Coumadin) for at least 3 weeks prior (and 4 weeks after) the procedure, to avoid the risk of an embolic stroke.

3. *Prevent thromboembolic complications.* Warfarin (Coumadin) prevents thromboembolism in high-risk patients, e.g., those with a prior TIA or stroke, valvular heart disease, CHF, hypertension, diabetes, and age 75 years. NOACS, e.g., dabigatran (Pradaxa), an oral direct thrombin inhibitor, and rivaroxaban (Xarelto), apixaban (Eliquis), and edoxaban (Savaysa), oral factor Xa inhibitors, are safe and effective alternatives to warfarin in patients with "nonvalvular" atrial fibrillation (i.e., without a mechanical valve or rheumatic MS) who have difficulty monitoring or controlling the PT/INR. Of note, aspirin, with or without clopidogrel (Plavix), is less effective than warfarin and the NOACs for the prevention of thromboembolic complications of atrial fibrillation.

4. *Consider AV nodal catheter ablation* with pacing for rate control, in patients refractory to medical therapy. *Radiofrequency (RF)* or *cryo ablation for cure* by circumferential isolation of foci ("triggers") in or around the pulmonary veins along with linear ablation in the LA may be considered for patients who fail or do not tolerate at least one antiarrhythmic drug or as first-line therapy for select patients with recurrent symptomatic paroxysmal atrial fibrillation.

The first step in managing the patient with atrial fibrillation is to decide whether there is a high likelihood of safe conversion to normal sinus rhythm or whether the patient should be allowed to remain in atrial fibrillation. The decision is governed by the risk of thromboembolism, the severity of symptoms, and whether the patient is likely to maintain sinus rhythm.

Urgent synchronized electrical cardioversion is indicated in patients with rapid atrial fibrillation who are hypotensive or have angina, CHF, or other evidence of severe hemodynamic compromise. In general, a patient with recent onset atrial fibrillation and no evidence of left atrial enlargement has a greater chance of achieving and maintaining normal sinus rhythm. If atrial fibrillation has been present for <48 hours, rate control (e.g., with beta blockers, calcium channel blockers, digoxin) along with electrical cardioversion can be performed. Patients with long-standing atrial fibrillation (especially if due to mitral valve disease, hypertension, or advanced LV dysfunction) are least likely to maintain normal sinus rhythm after cardioversion, but often have the most to gain if successful (due to the importance of "atrial kick" to cardiac output). Most patients, therefore, merit at least one attempt at cardioversion.

If the arrhythmia is long-standing, and the patient is not a suitable candidate for cardioversion, treatment should focus on ventricular rate control, and long-term stroke prophylaxis. Patients who have been in atrial fibrillation for >48 hours are more likely to have atrial thrombi and may develop embolic stroke (2–5% of cases) with immediate electrical or pharmacologic cardioversion. Restoration of atrial mechanical function, not DC shock, causes ejection of clot from the LA appendage. Keep in mind that atrial thrombi are not evident on transthoracic echo, but they can be seen on TEE. If atrial fibrillation is present for >48 hours, or the TEE reveals thrombi, therapeutic oral anticoagulation with warfarin (target INR 2-3) or NOAC is recommended ≥ 3 weeks before cardioversion, and at least 4 weeks after cardioversion is attempted, since the longer the atrial fibrillation is present, the longer the atria are mechanically stunned after cardioversion.

It is estimated that antiarrhythmic drugs (other than amiodarone) are only about 50% successful in maintaining sinus rhythm after one year. Amiodarone is effective at preventing recurrent atrial fibrillation in 50–75% of patients. All antiarrhythmic medications are accompanied by a risk of proarrhythmia, particularly in those with CHF. At the present time, it appears that both therapeutic strategies (i.e., rate control vs. maintaining sinus rhythm) are of equal benefit.

For patients with recurrent paroxysms of atrial fibrillation but no underlying heart disease (so-called "lone atrial fibrillation"), Class IC agents, e.g., flecainide (Tambocor) and propafenone (Rythmol) are safe and effective. Class III agents, e.g., sotalol (Betapace), amiodarone (Cordarone, Pacerone), and dofetilide (Tikosyn) are also effective but there is a risk of torsades de pointes, particularly with sotalol and dofetilide, in vulnerable patients. Overall, the incidence of torsades with amiodarone has been less than previously suspected. Cardioversion with maintenance of sinus rhythm by antiarrhythmic agents all have potentially serious side effects. Rate control with AV nodal blocking agents (e.g., beta blockers, rate-slowing calcium channel blockers, digoxin) should be given first. As mentioned above, accepting chronic atrial fibrillation with appropriate rate control and long-term anticoagulation is a viable option in many patients. Once atrial fibrillation is established as a persistent rhythm and the ventricular rate controlled, symptoms often subside. AV nodal blocking agents, however, should not be used if WPW is present, since conduction down the accessory pathway may be *enhanced* and fatal ventricular fibrillation may result.

Stroke risk should always be considered when contemplating anticoagulation. Patients ≤ 60 years of age with "lone" atrial fibrillation (i.e., no risk factors) have an excellent prognosis with an extremely low risk (~1%/year) for embolic phenomena. The risk of stroke in these patients is similar to the risk of serious bleed on anticoagulation. Therapy in this group, therefore, should be directed toward relief of symptoms with rate control as the primary objective. Some recommend aspirin therapy to such patients although no convincing data supports this approach.

On the basis of available information, it appears unlikely that most young patients with lone atrial fibrillation will benefit from chronic anticoagulation or antiarrhythmic therapy to prevent recurrences. In patients without structural heart disease, chemical conversion can be tried by using oral flecainide or propafenone as a one-dose trial ("pill in the pocket"). Chronic anticoagulation is indicated, however, in adults >60–65 years of age, particularly those who have additional stroke risk factors, e.g., CHF or LV systolic dysfunction, hypertension, diabetes, mitral valve disease, and history of prior embolic events, even if NSR is thought to be maintained since recurrent episodes of atrial fibrillation are often asymptomatic and can go undetected (i.e., "silent" atrial fibrillation). In patients with refractory symptomatic atrial fibrillation, or in those with persistently rapid rates, radiofrequency AV nodal ablation and permanent pacing may be considered. There is growing experience with RF ablation by circumferential isolation of foci ("triggers") in or around the pulmonary veins and linear ablation in the LA that initiate and perpetuate atrial fibrillation, following which sinus rhythm may be restored or maintained. Some patients with atrial fibrillation can be treated surgically to restore and maintain sinus rhythm by the "maze procedure", where multiple incisions are created in the atria to prevent reentry circuits at the time of cardiac surgery. To decrease stroke risk, obliteration of the LA appendage can be performed during the surgical "maze procedure". A percutaneous LA appendage occluder device, e.g., the Watchman, may be an effective alternative to reduce cardioembolic stroke in select patients with atrial fibrillation who are intolerant to anticoagulation.

Pearls:

- When evaluating the risk for stroke in atrial fibrillation, keep in mind the mnemonic "**CHADS-VASc**" (**C**HF, **H**ypertension, **A**ge ≥ 75, **D**iabetes, prior **S**troke or TIA, **V**ascular disease, **A**ge 65-74, and **S**ex **C**ategory [female]). Each risk factor is assigned 1 point except for prior stroke/TIA and age ≥ 75 years, which are assigned 2 points. Female sex adds to the score only when another risk factor is present. Anticoagulation is recommended for a score ≥ 2 (in men) and ≥ 3 (in women). Anticoagulation should be withheld for ~2-4 weeks after a large stroke, however, due to the risk of hemorrhagic conversion.

- When assessing the bleeding risk in atrial fibrillation, remember the mnemonic "**HAS-BLED**" (**H**ypertension, **A**bnormal renal/liver function, **S**troke, **B**leeding history or predisposition, **L**abile INR, **E**lderly [age >65], **D**rugs/Alcohol concomitantly [including antiplatelet agents and NSAIDs]).

- In patients with atrial fibrillation, "lenient" heart rate control (<110 beats/min at rest) may be as effective as "strict" heart rate control (<80 beats/min at rest) in preventing cardiovascular events.

- A narrow-complex supraventricular tachycardia (SVT) that has a regular heart rate of 150 beats/min is atrial flutter with 2:1 AV block, until proven otherwise.

- An irregularly irregular rhythm in a patient with COPD is more commonly *multifocal atrial tachycardia* (MAT) than atrial fibrillation. MAT is an irregular fast rhythm defined by the presence of three or more P waves of varying morphologies. It may also be caused by hypokalemia or hypomagnesemia. MAT occurs most commonly in chronic lung disease but is also seen in patients with severe metabolic abnormalities or sepsis. Potassium and magnesium replacement may suppress the tachycardia. Rate-slowing calcium channel blockers (e.g., verapamil) may be useful for rate control. Medications causing atrial irritability (e.g., theophylline, inhaled albuterol) should be avoided if possible. AV nodal ablation with permanent pacing can be helpful if refractory to medical treatment.

Supraventricular Tachycardias

Paroxysmal SVT occurs in individuals of all ages, and is often seen in otherwise healthy young adult females without underlying structural heart disease. *AV nodal reentrant tachycardia (AVNRT)* is the most common type of paroxysmal SVT, occurring in 50–60% of cases. The reentry circuit is located within the AV node with impulses traveling down the slow (α) pathway and then retrograde up the fast (β) pathway of the AV node. The atria and ventricles are depolarized simultaneously, and the P waves are hidden in the QRS complexes on the ECG. The episode usually begins and ends abruptly and may last seconds to several hours or longer. The QRS complexes are typically narrow.

AV reciprocating tachycardia (AVRT), which includes WPW, is the second most common form of paroxysmal SVT (30–40% of cases) and most commonly utilizes the normal AV pathway and an accessory bypass tract for antegrade and/ or retrograde conduction (preexcitation [WPW] syndrome). About one half of patients with the WPW pattern on a routine ECG have periodic tachyarrhythmias, whereas the other half demonstrate no rhythm disturbances. In some patients with this syndrome, the characteristic ECG features (short PR interval, delta wave) occurs intermittently, or not at all. In these patients, the accessory pathway functions only in the retrograde direction (i.e., "concealed"), so that the QRS complexes are electrocardiographically normal.

Frequently, the first episode of AVNRT occurs before the age of 30 although it may start after the patient has reached 60 years of age. AVNRT is characterized by the sudden onset and offset of a regular tachycardia at rates of 150 to 250 beats per minute. Many attacks of paroxysmal SVT resolve spontaneously. If not, vagal maneuvers (e.g., Valsalva maneuver [with leg elevation and supine positioning], carotid sinus massage, breath holding, immersing the face in ice water) may terminate the attack. *Response to vagal maneuvers may be diagnostic since paroxysmal SVT is, with rare exception, the only tachycardia that can be broken and stay normal during these maneuvers.* Adenosine (Adenocard), a naturally occurring nucleoside with a very short half life, is useful for the treatment of paroxysmal SVT. If adenosine is not effective in terminating AVNRT, or if acute bronchospasm is present, IV verapamil (or diltiazem) is generally effective. IV adenosine and verapamil are equally effective in rapidly terminating paroxysmal SVT in >90% of cases. Verapamil should not be used as a diagnostic test, however, because it may precipitate ventricular fibrillation (VF) if the initial rhythm is VT. *AV nodal blocking agents (e.g., adenosine, beta blockers, calcium channel blockers, and digoxin) should be avoided in WPW, because they can lead to arrhythmia acceleration through the accessory pathway.* Extremely rapid ventricular rates are possible and may precipitate hemodynamic collapse and sudden death. (**Note:** IV procainamide and ibutilide are the drugs of choice for controlling the rate of atrial fibrillation in patients with bypass tracts because they decrease conduction over the accessory pathway and are safe if antegrade accessory pathway conduction is present in atrial fibrillation.)

Prevention of frequent attacks of SVT can be achieved by beta blockers, calcium channel blockers (e.g., verapamil, diltiazem), and digoxin. Radiofrequency ablation of the abnormal reentrant circuit (or accessory pathway) has a >90% success rate. In atrial flutter, Class IA agents should not be given prior to the administration of AV nodal blocking agents, since 1:1 conduction through the AV node may result, thereby increasing the ventricular response.

A history of paroxysmal SVT in a young woman should lead you to consider three possibilities:

- SVT in an otherwise normal heart
- Underlying MVP
- The possibility of preexcitation (WPW) syndrome

When atrial fibrillation occurs with an extremely rapid ventricular response, consider the presence of an accessory pathway (as in WPW). Remember that abnormal Q waves can (and often are) mistaken as being caused by an acute MI in patients with WPW syndrome. When conduction occurs antegrade via the AV node and then returns retrograde up the accessory pathway, the QRS complexes during SVT appear normal and are not widened (so-called *orthodromic AV reentrant tachycardia*). When antegrade conduction is through the accessory pathway, and retrograde conduction is through the normal pathway, the QRS complexes are maximally preexcited, so that they appear bizarre and widened (so-called *antidromic reciprocating tachycardia*) and may be confused with VT. Such cases of retrograde conduction respond best to procainamide (which prolongs the refractory period of the accessory pathway) or to electrical cardioversion. As previously discussed, AV nodal blocking agents, e.g., digitalis, beta blocker, and verapamil (although useful in rapid atrial fibrillation in the absence of WPW) should be avoided in WPW, since they may shorten the refractory period in the accessory pathway, further increase the ventricular rate, and precipitate ventricular fibrillation. Worthy of mention, continuous supraventricular tachycardia may produce LV systolic dysfunction (tachycardia-induced cardiomyopathy). Medical and/or electrophysiological (i.e., radiofrequency catheter ablation) control of the tachycardia can cause reversal of the cardiomyopathy.

Ventricular Tachycardia

Ventricular tachycardia is defined as three or more consecutive PVCs. It may produce cardiac arrest, syncope, mildly symptomatic hypotension, or no symptoms other than the sensation of tachycardia. Although some forms of VT can occur in younger patients without structural heart disease, most VT is associated with serious underlying heart disease and is either nonsustained (lasting less than 30 seconds) or sustained (lasting more than 30 seconds). Common causes include myocardial ischemia, acute MI, dilated cardiomyopathy, hypertrophic cardiomyopathy, MVP, CHF, or digitalis toxicity. *Torsades de pointes*, a form of VT in which QRS morphology waxes and wanes ("twists") around the baseline, may occur spontaneously in hypokalemia or hypomagnesemia or after any drug that prolongs the QT interval. A wide complex tachycardia, usually between 140 and 220 beats/min on the ECG, along with AV dissociation, capture or fusion beats, and extreme axis deviation in a patient with underlying heart disease, acute ischemia, a history of MI, cardiomyopathy with a low EF, is a clue to VT, until proven otherwise. (**Note:** "Capture" beats are normal QRS complexes that appear amidst the wide, abnormal QRS complexes of VT, representing atrial waves that got through to the ventricles. A "fusion" beat is a QRS that partially appears, having fused with an abnormal QRS complex in VT. Both capture and fusion beats help confirm that the abnormal QRS complexes originate in the ventricles.) Unlike paroxysmal SVT, many episodes of VT do not stop spontaneously. Even worse, there is a predisposition for VT to deteriorate into ventricular fibrillation (VF).

Treatment is directed at ending the bout of VT. If the VT is acute and hemodynamically stable, IV amiodarone (Cordarone), procainamide (Pronestyl), or lidocaine (Xylocaine) can be used. If IV administered medications do not produce immediate results, or if the patient is hemodynamically unstable (i.e., hypotension, CHF, or angina is present), immediate synchronized electrical cardioversion should be employed. In acute MI, prophylactic lidocaine is associated with a higher rate of asystole and a poorer outcome and is no longer recommended, except in treating patients with non-sustained VT. The management of torsades de pointes differs from that of other forms of VT. Class I or III antiarrhythmic agents, which prolong the QT interval, should be avoided (or withdrawn immediately if being used). Beta blockers, IV magnesium, along with correction of electrolyte abnormalities, e.g., hypokalemia and/or temporary pacing, can both break and prevent the rhythm disturbance.

The next step in treatment of VT is to prevent it from recurring. Options include medication, correction of an underlying problem, use of an implantable device, or surgical or catheter ablation procedures to eliminate the site in the LV or RV that is causing the VT. In post-MI patients, there is movement away from the use of most of the antiarrhythmic agents for the suppression of ventricular arrhythmias because of the increased risk of proarrhythmia (e.g., torsades de pointes). Beta blockers, however, have a beneficial effect on long-term outcome and have evolved as the drugs of choice; amiodarone also has good evidence in its favor. Amiodarone can also induce polymorphic VT ("torsades de pointes") although

131

the drug has a lower incidence of pro-arrhythmic effects than other antiarrhythmic agents. Side effects (usually dose-related) of amiodarone include bluish-gray discoloration of the skin, thyroid dysfunction, pulmonary fibrosis (rarely, but occasionally irreversible), corneal microdeposits and liver abnormalities.

VT in the setting of acute ischemia or MI responds to treatment of the ischemia and does not necessarily require prolonged antiarrhythmic therapy. For chronic, recurrent, sustained VT, either implantable cardiac defibrillator (ICD) and/or antiarrhythmic therapy (guided by EPS studies) should be considered. A distinction must be made between suppression of PVCs (which is virtually useless) and control of VT or VF, which can prolong life. ICDs are most beneficial for patients with depressed LV function and life-threatening ventricular arrhythmias. Amiodarone is often used together with an ICD. Although the implanted device is the ultimate protection against sudden cardiac death, the drug prevents or reduces the number of serious arrhythmias that cause the device to fire, thus lengthening battery life and minimizing the psychological (and sometimes physical) effects of being "shocked" multiple times. Electrolyte abnormalities e.g., $\downarrow K^+$, $\downarrow Mg^{++}$ (particularly with torsades de pointes), digitalis toxicity or pacemaker malfunction can be the cause of VT, and should be kept in mind and treated accordingly.

If sudden cardiac death occurs in the patient with CAD in the absence of an MI, the prognosis is paradoxically worse than if in the setting of an MI (since it suggests active ongoing ischemia). Urgent cardiac catheterization (with an eye toward revascularization to prevent another event) is warranted. ICD is indicated for cardiac arrest due to VT/VF that is not due to a transient or reversible cause. Another cause of sudden cardiac death is *Brugada's syndrome*, an autosomal dominant disorder most frequently associated with mutations in the sodium channel (*SCN5A*), followed by the L-type calcium channel (*CACNA1C*) genes. In affected patients (most commonly young Asian males) with syncope or cardiac arrest (due to polymorphic VT/VF), the ECG reveals RBBB with ST segment elevation in precordial leads V1 and V2. Because antiarrhythmic drug therapy is thought to be ineffective, and the chance of recurrent syncope or sudden death is substantial (~35% within 24 months), implantation of an ICD is usually recommended for these patients.

Bradyarrhythmias and Conduction Abnormalities

Bradyarrhythmias are common, especially in young, athletic individuals. They are usually due to increased vagal tone and do not require intervention. Abnormalities of conduction can occur between the sinus node and atrium, within the AV node, and in the intraventricular conduction pathways. Bradyarrhythmias due to these abnormalities may occur with aging and are usually due to idiopathic fibrosis in the conduction tissue (*Lenegre's disease*) or calcification of the cardiac skeleton (*Lev's disease*), CAD, cardiac trauma (postcardiac surgery/TAVR), tumors, infections (endocarditis, Chagas, Lyme), or other inflammatory or infiltrative disease (e.g., amyloid, sarcoid). Abnormalities of the cardiac conduction system may result in three general clinical syndromes:

- The *sick sinus syndrome* (which includes marked sinus bradycardia, sinoatrial exit block or arrest, and the so-called brady-tachy syndrome)
- *AV nodal-His heart block*
- *Intraventricular (bundle branch) block*

Patients with bradyarrhythmias and conduction abnormalities may be asymptomatic, or present with syncope, near-syncope, lightheadedness, worsening CHF or angina.

For the most part, management of bradyarrhythmias and conduction disturbances involves:

- Excluding self-limited causes (e.g., inferior MI, which causes transient ischemia of the AV node).
- Withdrawing bradycardia-inducing drugs (e.g., digoxin, beta blockers, rate-slowing calcium channel blockers).
- Administering intravenous atropine sulfate (an anticholinergic agent that blocks the vagal effect and thereby increases heart rate and enhances AV nodal conduction), or temporary pacing, if symptoms, e.g., dizziness, near-syncope or syncope, and angina pectoris, as well as hypotension, or frequent PVCs (due to the slow rhythm) are present.
- Deciding on the need for implantation of a permanent pacemaker. Asymptomatic sinus bradycardia, first degree AV block, and Mobitz type I second degree AV block often need no specific therapy. The presence of asymptomatic bifascicular block is not an indication for pacemaker therapy. A pacemaker may especially be indicated in symptomatic Mobitz type II second degree AV block, third degree heart block, chronic bifascicular or trifascicular block, or sick sinus syndrome. A pacemaker may also be indicated when there is a need to continue bradycardia-inducing drugs for other conditions.

Chapter 21.   Dilated Cardiomyopathy

Cardiomyopathies are defined as diseases of the myocardium associated with mechanical and/or electrical dysfunction. Cardiomyopathies either are confined to the heart (primary) or are part of generalized systemic disorders (secondary). The traditional classification of cardiomyopathies divides them into three main groups:

1. *Dilated cardiomyopathy* (systolic dysfunction)
2. *Hypertrophic cardiomyopathy* (diastolic dysfunction)
3. *Restrictive (or obliterative) cardiomyopathy* (diastolic dysfunction) (e.g., amyloidosis, sarcoidosis, hemochromatosis, scleroderma)

Dilated cardiomyopathy, the most common form of cardiomyopathy, is characterized by LV or biventricular dilatation, impaired contractility, and systolic dysfunction. Symptoms and signs of CHF are common in patients with dilated cardiomyopathy. While some cases have specific known causes, many are idiopathic (of unknown cause). Specific secondary causes should be strongly entertained: in the clinical setting of a previous "flu-like" illness or other viral infection (e.g., parvo B19, human herpes 6, coxsackie, echo, human immunodeficiency virus [HIV]), CAD, heavy alcohol consumption, illicit drug use (e.g., cocaine), chemotherapy (e.g., doxorubicin [Adriamycin]), connective tissue diseases (e.g., periarteritis, systemic lupus erythematosus), the pregnant or postpartum state, thyroid disease (either hypo- or hyperthyroidism), sleep apnea, emotional or physical stress, or chronic persistent tachycardia (usually supraventricular). At present, most cases of cardiomyopathy are considered idiopathic, and presumed to be either familial (genetic) or an autoimmune response to a previous insult to the myocardium, most commonly (but not necessarily) viral. A relatively uncommon, but frequently overlooked cause of "idiopathic" dilated cardiomyopathy is LV hypertrabeculation/noncompaction (also called "spongy myocardium"), thought to be either a genetic (embryologic defect) or an acquired morphologic trait. It is important to exclude secondary causes, however, since certain conditions (e.g., CAD, alcohol, sleep apnea, thyroid disease, tachycardia or stress) may be "curable" or at least partially reversible.

The clinical course of dilated cardiomyopathy is often insidious, without any history of a precipitating factor (**Figure 21-1**).

Treatment of dilated cardiomyopathy consists of the standard approach to LV systolic dysfunction and includes *ACE inhibitors/ARBs or angiotensin receptor*

Figure 21-1

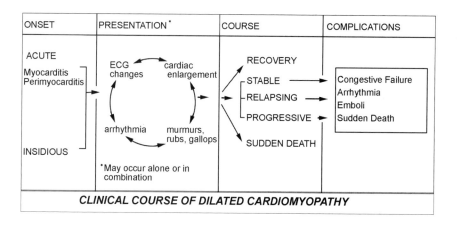

ONSET	PRESENTATION *	COURSE	COMPLICATIONS
ACUTE Myocarditis Perimyocarditis — INSIDIOUS —	ECG changes ↔ cardiac enlargement arrhythmia ↔ murmurs, rubs, gallops *May occur alone or in combination	RECOVERY STABLE RELAPSING PROGRESSIVE SUDDEN DEATH	Congestive Failure Arrhythmia Emboli Sudden Death

CLINICAL COURSE OF DILATED CARDIOMYOPATHY

neprilysin inhibitor (ARNI) (see below), *beta blockers, diuretics, digoxin, and aldosterone antagonists. Long term anticoagulation* with warfarin is advisable (if no contraindications exists) for patients with severe LV dysfunction, established or paroxysmal atrial fibrillation, a history of previous thromboembolism, or echo evidence of intracardiac thrombi, because of the high incidence of systemic and pulmonary embolization. Implantation of a cardioverter defibrillator has been shown to be more efficacious than antiarrhythmic drug therapy in patients with mild to moderate (NYHA class II-III) CHF and poor LV function (EF ≤35%), and those with sustained VT or sudden cardiac death (due to the proarrhythmic drug effects of antiarrhythmic drug therapy, i.e., potential to aggravate arrhythmias). Some patients with severe underlying CAD may have a significant amount of viable (stunned or hibernating) myocardium and may benefit from coronary artery bypass graft (CABG) surgery. Certain patients with advanced cardiomyopathy, particularly those with LBBB and a wide QRS complex ≥ 150 msec (which reflects LV dyssynchrony) may benefit from cardiac resynchronization therapy with biventricular pacing, which uses 3 leads: one lead in the right atrium, one in the right ventricle, and a third through the coronary sinus into a cardiac vein on the lateral wall of the left ventricle. Beneficial effects include reverse remodeling (decreased heart size and ventricular volumes, improved ejection fraction, and decreased mitral regurgitation). Other patients with end-stage disease and symptoms refractory to medical therapy may require cardiac transplantation. Implantable LV assist devices appear to have a role as a bridge to transplantation.

Dietary restriction of sodium is one of the most important aspects of treatment of a patient with congestive heart failure. It is also one of the most neglected. Many patients are told to "cut down" on salt, but no specific dietary education and counseling is provided. In fact, many patients say they're on a sodium-restricted diet but upon further questioning about where and what they ate, quickly identify no significant restriction at all. Beware of hidden sodium (e.g., in packaged, convenience, "fast", and canned foods). Advise your patients to be "heart-smart" and avoid eating such foods as pickles, chips and processed meats (e.g., ham, lunch meats). A "trick of the trade": You can tell that the patient is not adhering to a low-sodium diet if he or she states "The food 'tastes good' (i.e., contains too much salt) when I eat out (e.g., fast-food, delicatessen, Chinese or Italian restaurant)".

Mechanical heart support therapies, e.g., implantable LV assist devices, may also have a role as permanent or "destination" therapy. The prognosis for patients with dilated cardiomyopathy and advanced CHF is poor, with an average 5 year survival rate of <50%. The current 5 and 10 year survival rates after transplantation are ~75% and 55%, respectively. Because of the scarcity of donor hearts, however, fewer than 2500 transplants (out of the 20,000 patients who could potentially benefit) are performed in the United States each year.

Chapter 22. Hypertrophic Cardiomyopathy

Hypertrophic cardiomyopathy is a primary disorder of the heart muscle characterized by marked LV hypertrophy, with or without outflow tract obstruction, in the absence of an identifiable cause (e.g., hypertension, valvular AS). This chapter will review the pharmacologic approach to the patient with hypertrophic obstructive cardiomyopathy (HOCM) along with the risk factors for sudden cardiac death.

Management of HOCM

Hypertrophic obstructive cardiomyopathy previously called idiopathic hypertrophic subaortic stenosis [IHSS]) is a genetic heart muscle disease that occurs in about 1 out of 500 births. It is a common cause of sudden death in young athletes who die in the course of heavy exercise.

The outflow tract obstruction in HOCM is "dynamic", i.e., its magnitude may vary between examinations and even from beat to beat and can be provoked by pharmacologic interventions that reduce LV volume or chamber size (e.g., nitrates, diuretics) or enhance LV contractility (e.g., digitalis, other inotropic agents). Therefore, a history of worsening chest pain, shortness of breath, or syncope in a patient receiving these medications should alert the astute clinician to the diagnosis.

Medical treatment attempts to reduce the outflow tract obstruction, relax the ventricle, and avoid rhythm disturbances that may be associated with this condition:

- Beta blockers are the initial treatment of choice in symptomatic patients. Calcium channel blockers (e.g., verapamil) may also be useful in relieving symptoms (to allow more time for diastolic filling).

- If atrial fibrillation supervenes, every effort should be made to restore normal sinus rhythm (and preserve "atrial kick"). Frequent paroxysms or established atrial fibrillation indicate the need for long-term anticoagulation.

- Although at increased risk for infective endocarditis, recent guidelines no longer recommend antibiotic prophylaxis based solely on lifetime risk (see chapter 24).

- Certain anti-arrhythmic agents, e.g., disopyramide (due to its negative inotropic effects) and amiodarone, may be effective forms of therapy.

- Avoid nitrates, diuretics, digitalis, and other inotropic agents as they increase LV outflow tract gradient and worsen symptoms.

Surgical relief of the outflow tract gradient by myotomy and myectomy of the hypertrophied septum (when symptoms persist despite intensive pharmacologic treatment), or mitral valve replacement (reserved for the few in whom severe MR develops) provide mechanical solutions to the problem of dynamic LV outflow tract obstruction. In experienced hands, myectomy has a low operative mortality (~1–2%) and most patients have long-lasting improvement in their clinical outcome. Percutaneous transcoronary septal reduction with alcohol, along with dual chamber pacing (to reduce outflow tract gradient), and implantable cardioverter defibrillators (ICDs) may also be considered in the treatment strategy, and now provide additional forms of therapy for those patients who are refractory to medical therapy. The ICD is the most reliable and effective treatment for patients at high risk, particularly those who survive a cardiac arrest. Long-term results of these newer procedures, however, are under investigation. Recent studies have cast doubt on the value of dual chamber pacing and suggest that improvement is often largely due to a placebo effect. Furthermore, follow-up of patients after septal ablation is relatively brief and there is some concern that the permanent scar produced within the septum may eventually generate serious rhythm disturbances and actually increase risk for sudden death.

Risk of Sudden Death

The most alarming aspect of this disease is the risk of sudden death. Unlike with valvular AS, reduction or abolition of the systolic pressure gradient across the obstruction (by surgical or other treatments) does not abolish this risk. Analyses suggest that the risk of sudden death is not as high as previously believed, only ~1% per year. The risk of sudden cardiac death increases in patients with malignant ventricular arrhythmias, syncope, a family history of sudden death, severe LV hypertrophy (≥30 mm), high risk mutations, a blunted or hypotensive blood pressure response to exercise, and is more common in children and young adults (particularly athletes). The presence of a resting LV outflow tract gradient of ≥ 30 mmHg in patients with HOCM is a strong independent predictor of progression to severe symptoms of CHF and/or death. Although symptoms due to outflow obstruction may be relieved by drugs with negative inotropic properties (e.g., beta blockers, verapamil, disopyramide), these agents do not prevent sudden arrhythmic death. Patients with malignant ventricular arrhythmias and unexplained syncope in the presence of a positive family history for sudden death are probably best managed with an ICD. Since sudden cardiac death (due to ventricular tachyarrhythmias) usually occurs during heavy exertion, patients with HOCM should not participate in any strenuous exercise or high-intensity competitive sports. First-degree relatives of an affected individual should undergo periodic clinical screening with ECG and echo (since the timing of onset of HOCM is variable), along with genetic testing, if a definite pathogenic mutation has been identified.

Chapter 23. Valvular Heart Disease

Valvular heart disease (VHD) is one of the major types of cardiac disease encountered in clinical practice. There are five steps the practitioner should take in the clinical evaluation of the patient with VHD.

- Correctly diagnosing the affected valve (s)
- Estimating the severity of the lesion
- Judging its effect on the myocardium
- Deciding the need (or lack thereof) for infective endocarditis (and/or antistreptococcal) prophylaxis
- Deciding on the advisability and/or timing of surgical (or catheter-based) intervention

*Note: Antibiotic prophylaxis is no longer recommended for patients with VHD unless the patient has a history of previous endocarditis, or has undergone a valve replacement or repair using prosthetic material.

AORTIC STENOSIS (AS)

Aortic stenosis (AS) is the most common fatal valvular heart lesion in adults. In the older population (i.e., those over 65 years of age), "degenerative" calcification of a normal trileaflet aortic valve (aortic sclerosis), now considered to be an inflammatory process related to atherosclerosis, has emerged as the most common cause. Younger adults (particularly males) with isolated aortic stenosis most often have a congenitally bicuspid valve traumatized by abnormal turbulent flow patterns, which over years to decades produced fibrosis and calcification by a process of "wear and tear". Rheumatic heart disease may also cause AS but is infrequent without associated mitral valve involvement.

Management of AS

The question of surgical intervention in asymptomatic patients with significant AS remains controversial. The asymptomatic patient with valvular AS may generally be treated medically until symptoms develop. The risk of sudden death in asymptomatic patients is extremely low (<1%). Patients should be advised to report the onset of symptoms as soon as they occur. Once symptoms of angina, syncope, or CHF develop, survival is likely limited to 5 years, 3 years, or 2 years, respectively, unless surgery is performed. Aortic valve replacement in the symptomatic patient with significant valvular AS, therefore, should be strongly recommended without delay.

While "watchful waiting" is generally considered safe in asymptomatic patients with valvular AS, some experts suggest that asymptomatic patients with critical AS (aortic valve area < 0.6 cm^2, mean gradient > 60 mmHg) and an expected low operative risk (<1%), and those who have LV dysfunction (EF <50%), develop symptoms or hypotension during closely supervised exercise testing, or have a high likelihood of rapid progression (e.g., age, severe calcification, CAD) may benefit from surgery.

Although vasodilator therapy has become the mainstay of treatment for patients with CHF, these agents can produce hypotension, syncope, and even death in a patient with severe aortic stenosis in the setting of a fixed cardiac output and, thus, are best avoided. The possibility of halting the progression of aortic valve sclerosis (along with CAD) with lipid-lowering therapy ("statins") is an intriguing but as yet unproven prospect for the management of this disease. Operative mortality rate in elective surgery is ~3–5% and increases with age and with worsening hemodynamic status. The overall response to aortic valve replacement is excellent. If LV function is depressed, an improvement can be anticipated after surgery once the obstruction is relieved.

In general, a mechanical prosthesis is recommended if the patient is young or middle-aged, and if there is no reason to withhold anticoagulation. A bioprosthetic tissue valve from a human (homograft) or animal (heterograft, e.g., porcine, bovine pericardial) is recommended for older patients (>75 years of age) with limited life expectancy, bleeding tendency, or anticipated difficulty with anticoagulation (i.e., warfarin). Lifelong anticoagulation with warfarin is required for mechanical prostheses but is not essential with bioprosthesis after the first 3 months (unless additional risk factors for emboli, e.g., atrial fibrillation, LV dysfunction, previous thromboembolism, are present). Approximately 30–50% of heterograft valves need replacing within 10 years after implantation. Some centers have begun performing the *Ross procedure*, which entails switching the patient's pulmonary valve to the aortic position and placing a bioprosthesis in the pulmonary position, since they do not deteriorate as fast on the right side of the heart. Percutaneous balloon valvotomy for AS is not the preferred approach because improvement in aortic valve area is limited (frequently <1 year) due to a high incidence of restenosis. It may be useful, however, as a temporary measure, in patients with serious severe comorbidity, patients requiring urgent noncardiac surgery, and as a bridge to AVR in hemodynamically unstable patients with cardiogenic shock or severe CHF. Although patients with valvular AS are at increased risk for developing infective endocarditis, recent guidelines no longer recommend prophylactic antibiotics before dental and other invasive procedures unless there is a past history of endocarditis or prior prosthetic valve replacement. Patients with degenerative calcific AS have an increased incidence of lower GI bleeding, often related to right-sided colonic angiodysplasia (Heyde's syndrome). AVR in these patients often prevents recurrent bleeding.

Presently, the risks of surgery and prosthetic valve complications in the asymptomatic patient with normal LV function outweigh the benefits of preventing sudden cardiac death and prolonging survival. Asymptomatic patients with severe valvular AS and declining LV function (EF < 50%), or those with moderate-severe AS undergoing CABG or surgery on the aorta or another heart valve, should be considered for aortic valve replacement. The surgical mortality is acceptable (~10%) among elderly patients and those with concurrent LV systolic dysfunction. Transcatheter aortic valve replacement (TAVR) is a viable alternative to surgery for intermediate to high risk or inoperable patients with severe symptomatic AS. Keep in mind that as surgical and percutaneous techniques continue to improve, patients with significant AS may become candidates for valve replacement earlier in the course of the disease.

AORTIC REGURGITATION

Chronic AR

There are multiple etiologies for chronic aortic regurgitation (AR). In an age of declining incidence of rheumatic fever and syphilis, degenerative disorders of the aortic root and cusps are the most common causes. AR frequently results from dilatation of the ascending aorta (ascending aortic aneurysm, cystic medial necrosis of the aorta, aortic dissection) and/or severe long-standing hypertension. Pure AR may be due to primary valve disease (bicuspid aortic valve, calcific degeneration, endocarditis, rheumatic). It can also be caused by rheumatoid arthritis, ankylosing spondylitis, and systemic lupus erythematosus. Recent studies have shown an association between the use of weight reduction drugs (*Phen-Fen*) and an increased prevalence of AR.

Acute AR

Acute AR can result from aortic dissection, infective endocarditis or trauma.

Management of Chronic and Acute AR

AR can be treated either medically or surgically, depending on the acuteness of presentation, symptoms, and LV size and function.

If hypertension is present in patients with chronic AR, treatment with afterload reducing agents (e.g., dihydropyridine calcium channel blockers, ACE inhibitors/ARBs, hydralazine) should be initiated. Theoretically, beta-blockers should be avoided, because they slow the heart rate, prolong diastole, and thus may worsen

AR. Vasodilator therapy (ACE inhibitors/ARBs) along with the cautious use of beta-blockers (which may exert beneficial effects on LV dilatation and remodeling) may be considered, however, in symptomatic patients with severe AR, those with LV systolic dysfunction (to improve hemodynamics before proceeding with AVR), and those who are not surgical candidates (because of comorbidities).

Data on the benefits of medical treatment in asymptomatic severe AR are controversial. There are no recommendations for vasodilator therapy in patients with severe, chronic AR who are asymptomatic with normal LV systolic function and have no hypertension.

Beta-blockers (by reducing aortic wall stress) and vasodilating agents, e.g., ARBs (by blocking TGF-beta) may slow the rate of aortic dilatation in patients with Marfan's syndrome.

Although at increased risk for acquiring infective endocarditis, antibiotic prophylaxis is no longer recommended in patients with AR unless there is a previous history of endocarditis. Asymptomatic patients with normal LV function may participate in all kinds of activities. However, strenuous isometric exercise should be avoided.

Aortic valve replacement is advised in patients with chronic AR when symptoms appear, the ejection fraction is <50%, the LV end-systolic dimension is >50 mm or the end-diastolic dimension is >65 mm on echo (if surgical risk is low). Early LV dysfunction will probably reverse with aortic valve replacement. AR due to aortic root disease requires repair or replacement of the root as well as the aortic valve (Bentall procedure), which is a more difficult operation.

At present, transcatheter aortic valve replacement (TAVR) is not approved for use in the U.S. in patients with native AR (due to concerns over the lack of valvular calcification that may prevent secure anchoring). Transcatheter "valve-in-valve" replacement, or insertion of a vascular plug (occluder device), however, may be an option in anatomically suitable patients with bioprosthetic paravalvular AR.

Because of the embolic and anticoagulation risks of prosthetic aortic valves, the goal is to delay surgery without subjecting the patient to an irreversible loss of LV function. At the present time, it seems prudent to intervene surgically as soon as asymptomatic patients demonstrate a clear, persistent deterioration in LV function (even if mild). Following surgery, LV size usually decreases and LV function improves, except when dysfunction has been present chronically.

Acute AR can be catastrophic. In patients with acute AR, prompt recognition, appropriate antibiotic therapy (if infective endocarditis is the cause), and emergent surgical intervention (in patients with acute AR due to dissection or trauma and/or who are hemodynamically unstable) can be lifesaving.

MITRAL REGURGITATION (MR)

With the decline of rheumatic fever, MVP has become the most common cause of valvular mitral regurgitation (MR) (~65% of cases).

Management of Chronic MR

Mild-to-moderate MR usually causes no symptoms and has an excellent prognosis unless infective endocarditis or spontaneous chordal rupture occurs. Although patients with MR are at increased risk for acquiring infective endocarditis, recent guidelines no longer recommend routine antibiotic prophylaxis, unless there is a history of previous endocarditis or prior prosthetic valve replacement/repair. Congestive symptoms are improved with dietary restriction of sodium, along with diuretics and vasodilator therapy (e.g., ACE inhibitors/ARBs). There are no long-term studies to indicate that vasodilators are beneficial in asymptomatic patients with normal LV function. Atrial fibrillation is a late occurrence (usually denotes marked LA enlargement) and requires rate control (with beta blockers, calcium channel blockers, digitalis) and anticoagulation therapy with warfarin (to achieve a target INR of 2-3). Electrical cardioversion is rarely successful on a long-term basis.

Because progressive and irreversible deterioration of LV function may occur prior to the onset of symptoms, early operation is indicated even in asymptomatic patients with chronic MR when the ejection fraction is declining ($\leq 60\%$) or LV dilation (end systolic dimension ≥ 40 mm on echo) is present. Surgical intervention should be considered when symptoms develop as long as the ejection fraction is >30% and/or the LV end systolic dimension is <55mm. **Note:** An ejection fraction of <30% indicates severely reduced LV function. The ejection fraction should normally be $\geq 65\%$ in MR.) The onset of atrial fibrillation or pulmonary hypertension (PA pressure >50mmHg) is also an indication for surgery. With improved surgical techniques, mitral valve repair (valvuloplasty) now is being performed earlier (and in preference to valve replacement) than in the past, as the operative risk is lower and LV function better preserved when the subvalvular structures can be maintained intact after surgery. Advances in mitral valve surgery (including minimally invasive and robotically assisted valve repair and valve replacement with chordal preservation) have improved perioperative and longterm outcomes in patients with MR. Percutaneous approaches to valve repair, e.g., the edge-to-edge mitral clip, can be considered when the LV ejection fraction is <30% and the operative risk is high. However, due to the high incidence of residual MR, surgical repair (if feasible) remains the intervention of choice in patients who are acceptable candidates for operation.

Acute MR

Acute MR (caused by spontaneous chordae tendineae rupture, infective endocarditis, or papillary muscle rupture in the setting of acute MI) is a potentially lethal condition characterized by the abrupt onset of pulmonary edema and severe perfusion failure.

Because the patient with acute severe MR tolerates the lesion poorly, immediate surgical repair may be required following stabilization with inotropic agents, vasodilators (if tolerated), and IABP counterpulsation.

MITRAL VALVE PROLAPSE (MVP)

The most common mitral valve abnormality is mitral valve prolapse (MVP), affecting up to 2 to 3% of the population.

Management of Mitral Valve Prolapse (MVP)

Severe MVP (with valve leakage) is the most common heart condition associated with infective endocarditis. Endocarditis may also occur in the milder forms of MVP. Although MVP is the most common underlying condition that predisposes to the acquisition of infective endocarditis, the absolute incidence of endocarditis for the entire population with MVP is extremely low. Furthermore, MVP is not usually associated with the highest risk of an adverse outcome from infective endocarditis as are other higher risk cardiac conditions. Thus routine antibiotic prophylaxis is no longer recommended in these patients when undergoing dental, GI, or GU tract procedures (see chapter 24).

Beta blockers may be tried in symptomatic patients (e.g., palpitations, chest pain, and anxiety or panic attacks). Sudden death (most often caused by ventricular arrhythmias) is a rare occurrence. Most patients with MVP (~90%) have neither symptoms nor a high-risk profile. Patients with MVP should be reassured that their prognosis is generally excellent. The incidence of complications is very low and is usually associated with an increase in mitral valve leaflet thickness or hemodynamically significant MR. In general, complications increase with age and are more common in males than in females. Often, quiet reassurance of the benign prognosis and explanation of the disease entity is all that is required.

Patients with severe MR unresponsive to drug therapy, e.g., afterload reduction (ACE inhibitors, hydralazine and nitrates), may require valve repair and/or replacement. Restriction from competitive sports may be required for patients with MVP who have significant MR with LV enlargement and/or dysfunction, uncontrolled tachyarrhythmias, prolonged QT intervals, a history of unexplained syncope, aortic root enlargement, and a family history of sudden cardiac death.

RHEUMATIC MITRAL STENOSIS (MS)

Rheumatic fever is the major cause of mitral stenosis. Although we witnessed a dramatic decline in acute rheumatic fever in the United States (due to control of group A streptococcal infection), strep infections and acute rheumatic fever have recently re-emerged as clinical problems.

Management of Rheumatic Mitral Stenosis (MS)

- Preventive measures against rheumatic fever, including administration of either penicillin (or sulfadiazine or erythromycin, if allergic), are suggested in all patients for at least 10 years after the last RF episode, or until age 40 in those patients with frequent exposure to streptococcal infection, e.g., teachers and day-care workers. Recent guidelines, however, no longer recommended prophylactic antibiotics against infective endocarditis. Patients with MS should be managed medically unless symptoms persist despite such therapy.

- Systemic thromboembolism is a serious complication of MS, and anti-coagulation should be strongly considered in these patients (especially those with atrial fibrillation).

- Rate control (e.g., beta blockers, calcium channel blockers, digoxin) is indicated for atrial fibrillation. Electrical cardioversion should be attempted.

- Correction usually requires surgical intervention (valve replacement), but percutaneous balloon valvuloplasty may be considered a treatment option in symptomatic patients with MS and an orifice area of ≤ 1.5 cm^2 if they have suitable mitral valve morphology on echo, i.e., thin, mobile, noncalcified leaflets, with little subvalvular involvement (favorable "Wilkins score"), and minimal or no MR and no LA clot. Problems associated with prosthetic valves include thrombosis, perivalvular leak, endocarditis, and degenerative changes in tissue valves.

Tips regarding indications for valve surgery:

- In hemodynamically significant *valvular AS* (valve area ≤ 1.0 cm^2), it's time to operate once symptoms of CHF, syncope or angina develop. Surgery may be considered in asymptomatic patients when LV dysfunction (LV ejection fraction <50%) or an adverse response to exercise is present.

- In patients with *chronic AR*, consider surgery when symptoms (dyspnea, angina) develop or when objective signs of LV dilatation and/or dysfunction (LV ejection fraction <50% or LV end-systolic dimension >50 mm or LV end-diastolic dimension >65 mm) are present.

- In patients with *chronic MR* consider valve repair or replacement for symptoms or decline of LV function into the low-normal range (LV end systolic dimension ≥ 40 mm or ejection fraction 30-60%), or if new onset atrial fibrillation or pulmonary hypertension (PA pressure > 50mmHg) is present.

- In patients with severe *rheumatic MS* (valve area ≤ 1.5 cm^2), consider mitral balloon valvuloplasty (if pliable, noncalcified valve) or valve replacement if symptoms or pulmonary hypertension is present.

TRICUSPID REGURGITATION (TR)

Organic tricuspid valve disease may result from various etiologies including rheumatic heart disease, infectious endocarditis, myxomatous degeneration, metastatic carcinoid, tumor, RV infarction (papillary muscle rupture), severe blunt trauma, and right atrial myxoma. Significant "functional" tricuspid regurgitation (TR) may also result from pulmonary hypertension of any cause or RV failure.

Management of TR

Although patients with TR caused by an abnormal tricuspid valve are at increased risk for infective endocarditis, as with other forms of valvular heart disease, recent guidelines no longer recommend prophylactic antibiotics based solely on lifetime risk (see chapter 24). The basic principle of management of TR is to treat the underlying condition (e.g., infective endocarditis, cardiomyopathy, pulmonary hypertension). TR may decrease in severity if appropriate medical therapy improves global or right heart function, or results in a decrease in pulmonary artery pressure or resistance. Surgical intervention is usually unnecessary for primary organic TR without pulmonary hypertension. If TR is severe and refractory, valve repair or annuloplasty may be indicated and is often preferable to valve replacement. In the patient with mitral and/or aortic valve disease requiring valve surgery, decisions regarding the state of tricuspid valve function and the need for tricuspid annuloplasty or valve repair may require intraoperative transesophageal echocardiography (TEE).

Chapter 24.   Infective Endocarditis

Infective endocarditis occurs when infective organisms invade the endothelial (particularly the valvular) surfaces of the heart, causing tissue destruction and vegetations. Despite medical and surgical advances, the mortality rates remain high. This may be due to the fact that infective endocarditis is now occurring in older individuals, in patients unaware of having heart valve disease, in those with prosthetic valves or other intracardiac devices, and is being caused by aggressive organisms, e.g., staphylococci. This chapter will review the treatment and prevention of this complex, commonly missed, and potentially lethal disease.

Therapy and Prevention of Infective Endocarditis

Antibiotic therapy in patients with suspected infective endocarditis should begin after at least 3 sets of blood cultures are obtained. Empiric therapy should cover the most likely pathogens, including streptococci, staphylococci, enterococci and HACEK group. Pathogen directed therapy should be initiated once the causative organism has been identified. Prolonged intravenous antimicrobial therapy (for 4 to 6 weeks or longer) may be needed to eradicate the infection, sterilize the vegetation, and prevent recurrence. Valve replacement is often indicated when a staph aureus or fungal infection is present, a prosthetic valve is infected, complications (e.g., myocardial abscess or acute valvular dysfunction associated with CHF) has developed, medical therapy has failed, or a large vegetation or more than one embolic event has occurred (**Figure 24-1**). Device-related (pacemaker/ICD) endocarditis generally requires removal of the entire system, including the leads, with reimplantation, if needed, on the contralateral side.

For decades, it has been a commonly held belief that antimicrobial prophylaxis before procedures that may cause transient bacteremia can prevent infective endocarditis in patients at increased risk for this disorder. The effectiveness of this common practice, however, has never been established by controlled trials in humans. Experts now believe that infective endocarditis is much more likely to develop secondary to random bacteremias associated with daily activities, e.g., chewing food, brushing teeth, and flossing, than from transient bacteremia caused by a dental, gastrointestinal (GI) or genitourinary (GU) tract procedure. Furthermore, even if antimicrobial prophylaxis were 100% effective, it would only prevent an exceedingly small number of cases of infective endocarditis. In addition,

Figure 24-1

PHARMACOLOGIC APPROACH TO INFECTIVE ENDOCARDITIS

Antibiotic therapy for 4–6 weeks. Empiric therapy (before culture results available) in acutely ill patients: Native valve bacterial endocarditis (vancomycin is an appropriate choice for initial therapy in most). Prosthetic valve endocarditis (vancomycin + gentamycin + cefipime or a carbapenem with antipseudomonal activity, e.g., imipenem). As soon as possible, the empiric drug regimen should be adjusted based on culture results. Surgery for refractory CHF, persistent or refractory infection, worsening conduction defect, prosthetic valve malfunction or dehiscence, or staph aureus infection, recurrent emboli, fungal infection.

---

the risk of antibiotic-associated adverse events would exceed the benefit, if any, from the use of antibiotics.

Accordingly, the American Heart Association has issued updated guidelines on the prevention of infective endocarditis. Whereas previous guidelines recommended prophylaxis for individuals at increased lifetime risk for acquiring infective endocarditis, the revised guidelines emphasize prophylaxis only for patients with cardiac conditions associated with the highest risk for adverse outcome from infective endocarditis. "High risk" patients include those with prosthetic heart valves (including transcatheter valves) or prosthetic material used for valve repair; previous infective endocarditis; unrepaired, recently repaired (within 6 months), or partially repaired cyanotic congenital heart disease; and cardiac valvulopathy following heart transplantation.

Even for these "high risk" patients, prophylaxis is recommended only before dental procedures that involve manipulation of gingival tissue, or the periapical region of teeth, or perforation of the oral mucosa; invasive respiratory tract procedures involving incision or biopsy of the respiratory mucosa; or surgical procedures that involve infected skin or musculoskeletal structures. Infective endocarditis prophylaxis is no longer recommended for GU or GI tract procedures, even in these high risk patients. Antibiotic prophylaxis is also not recommended for other common procedures including ear and body piercing, tattooing, vaginal delivery, and hysterectomy.

Since the revised guidelines no longer recommend antimicrobial prophylaxis solely to prevent infective endocarditis, patients with MVP and mitral regurgitation or thickened valve leaflets, a congenital bicuspid aortic valve, calcific AS, rheumatic heart disease, or structural disorders, e.g., VSD and HOCM, are no longer considered candidates for prophylaxis. Routine prophylaxis is also not recommended prior to cardiac catheterization, or in patients with cardiac pacemakers, implanted defibrillators, coronary stents, or in those who have had CABG surgery. Although dental disease may increase the risk of infective endocarditis, the revised guidelines shift emphasis away from antimicrobial prophylaxis for dental procedures to meticulous oral health and hygiene and improved dental care in patients with conditions that carry an increased risk for the infection.

The revised (and somewhat controversial) prophylaxis recommendations are given in **Figures 24-2 to 24-4**.

148

Figure 24-2

ENDOCARDITIS PROPHYLAXIS IS RECOMMENDED FOR:

Cardiac Conditions*

- Prosthetic cardiac valves (including transcatheter valves) or prosthetic material used for valve repair
- Previous endocarditis
- Unrepaired, recently repaired (within 6 months), or partially repaired cyanotic congenital heart disease
- Cardiac valvulopathy following heart transplantation

Procedures

- Dental procedures that involve manipulation of gingival tissue or the periapical region of teeth or perforation of the oral mucosa (e.g., teeth extractions and cleanings)
- Invasive respiratory tract procedures involving incision or biopsy of the respiratory mucosa (e.g., tonsillectomy and adenoidectomy)
- Surgical procedures that involve infected skin or musculoskeletal structures

---

Adapted from Wilson W, Taubert, KA, Gewitz, M, et al. Prevention of Infective Endocarditis. Guidelines from the American Heart Association. A Guideline from the American Heart Association Rheumatic Fever, Endocarditis, and Kawasaki Disease Committee, Council on Cardiovascular Disease in the Young, and the Council on Clinical Cardiology, Council on Cardiovascular Surgery and Anesthesia, and the quality of Care and Outcomes Research Interdisciplinary Working Group. Circulation 115: 2007.

*Note: Antimicrobial prophylaxis is recommended only in patients with cardiac conditions associated with the highest risk of adverse outcome from endocarditis, not in patients solely at increased risk of acquiring infective endocarditis.

Figure 24-3

INFECTIVE ENDOCARDITIS PROPHYLAXIS IS NOT RECOMMENDED FOR:

Cardiac Conditions
- Mitral valve prolapse with mitral regurgitation or leaflet thickening
- Bicuspid aortic valve
- Rheumatic or acquired valvular heart disease
- Hypertrophic obstructive cardiomyopathy
- Atrial Septal Defect (ASD), Ventricular Septal Defect (VSD), and Patent Ductus Arteriosus (PDA)
- Cardiac catheterization, including PCI
- Coronary stents, cardiac pacemakers, implanted defibrillators
- Coronary artery disease or previous coronary bypass surgery

Procedures*
- Dental procedures that involve routine anesthetic injections through non-infected tissue, taking dental radiographs, placement of removable prosthodontic or orthodontic appliances, adjustment of orthodontic appliances, placement of orthodontic brackets, shedding of deciduous teeth, and bleeding from trauma to the lips or oral mucosa
- Bronchoscopy (without incision or biopsy of respiratory tract mucosa)
- GU (e.g., cystoscopy, urethral dilatation) or GI tract procedures, including endoscopy or colonoscopy
- Ear and body piercing, and tattooing
- Vaginal delivery and hysterectomy

Adapted from Wilson W, Taubert, KA, Gewitz, M, et al. Prevention of Infective Endocarditis. Guidelines from the American Heart Association. A Guideline from the American Heart Association Rheumatic Fever, Endocarditis, and Kawasaki Disease Committee, Council on Cardiovascular Disease in the Young, and the Council on Clinical Cardiology, Council on Cardiovascular Surgery and Anesthesia, and the quality of Care and Outcomes Research Interdisciplinary Working Group. Circulation 115: 2007.

*Note: In the case of a procedure that involves infected tissues, it may be necessary to provide appropriate doses of antibiotics for treatment of the established infection.

Figure 24-4

ENDOCARDITIS PROPHYLAXIS REGIMENS

Situation	Agent (single dose 30-60 min before procedure)
Oral prophylaxis	Amoxicillin*
Parenteral prophylaxis	Ampicillin or Cefazolin or Ceftriaxone or Clindamycin

---

***Note:** For penicillin-allergic individuals, cephalexin, cefadroxil, clindamycin, or azithromycin-clarithromycin may be used. Cephalosporins should not be used, however, in those with immediate-type hypersensitivity reaction (e.g., urticaria, angioedema, or anaphylaxis) to penicillin.

Adapted from Wilson W, Taubert, KA, Gewitz, M, et al. Prevention of Infective Endocarditis. Guidelines from the American Heart Association. A Guideline from the American Heart Association Rheumatic Fever, Endocarditis, and Kawasaki Disease Committee, Council on Cardiovascular Disease in the Young, and the Council on Clinical Cardiology, Council on Cardiovascular Surgery and Anesthesia, and the quality of Care and Outcomes Research Interdisciplinary Working Group. Circulation 115: 2007.

Chapter 25. Aortic and Peripheral Arterial Disease

Diseases of the aorta and its branches may present as one of three clinical conditions: *aortic dissection, aortic aneurysm, and peripheral arterial disease*. This chapter will discuss the management of these common vascular diseases.

Aortic Dissection

Acute *aortic dissection* and its variants, *intramural hematoma* and *penetrating atherosclerotic ulcer*, are part of a spectrum of acute, life-threatening aortic events termed *"acute aortic syndromes."*

- *Type A* dissections originate in the ascending aorta, usually within a few centimeters of the aortic valve, and either extend around the aortic arch into the descending aorta (type 1) or are limited to the ascending aorta (type 2).
- *Type B* (or type 3) dissections (which are less common than Type A) involve only the descending aorta and originate just distal to the origin of the left subclavian artery. Type B dissections have the best prognosis. **(Figure 25-1)**.

Surgical consultation should be obtained as soon as aortic dissection is suspected.

- For patients with proximal dissection, the immediate goal of treatment is to lower BP, first with IV beta blocker therapy, e.g., esmolol, labetalol (which also reduces shear stress by lowering the BP) and then with IV nitroprusside, while awaiting emergent surgical repair. *Misdiagnosis of aortic dissection as acute MI can have disastrous consequences should the patient receive anticoagulants or thrombolytic therapy.* Thrombolytic therapy can lead to exsanguination in this setting, and is therefore contraindicated. Pericardial tamponade may result and is generally a terminal event.
- For type A dissection, the ascending aorta and, if necessary, the aortic valve and arch are replaced with reimplantation of the coronary and brachiocephalic vessels. Aspirin, heparin, and thrombolytics are contraindicated. Following successful surgery, chronic beta blocker therapy and annual imaging (CT scan or MRI) are indicated to evaluate for the development of progressive aortic dilatation or recurrent dissection.

Figure 25-1

MAJOR TYPES OF AORTIC DISSECTION

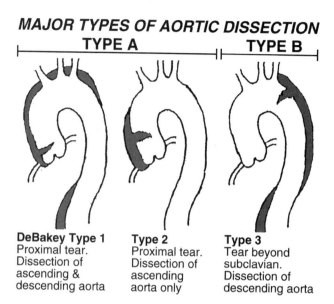

TYPE A		TYPE B

DeBakey Type 1
Proximal tear.
Dissection of
ascending &
descending aorta

Type 2
Proximal tear.
Dissection of
ascending
aorta only

Type 3
Tear beyond
subclavian.
Dissection of
descending aorta

- For type B (distal) dissection, long term pharmacologic therapy with beta blockers (or, if contraindicated, verapamil or diltiazem) is recommended as long as the patient remains stable. Surgical treatment, after several weeks of pharmacologic therapy, is advised by some authorities who believe that the majority of type B dissections will ultimately develop an indication for surgical intervention, e.g., increasing aortic size, an enlarging saccular aneurysm, compromise of major branches of the aorta, or symptoms related to their chronic dissection. Catheter-based repair with endovascular stent-grafts is currently being employed as an alternative to surgery.

Aortic Aneurysm

An *aortic aneurysm* is a localized ≥50% dilatation ("bulge") of the aorta involving all three layers of the vessel wall (intima, media, adventitia). The most common location for aneurysm formation is the infrarenal abdominal aorta, followed by the ascending thoracic aorta. Ascending thoracic aortic aneurysms (TAAs) are generally caused by cystic medial necrosis (as may be seen in Marfan's, LoeysDietz, and Ehlers-Danlos syndromes, bicuspid aortic valve, aortitis, and hypertension), whereas abdominal aortic aneurysms (AAAs) are primarily associated with atherosclerosis and its risk factors, i.e., advanced age, hypertension, smoking, dyslipidemia, male gender, and family history. The pathogenesis of AAA involves a

153

combination of inflammation, a proteolytic breakdown in the structural proteins elastin and collagen, and biochemical stresses which lead to weakening of the vessel wall.

Unstable patients with a ruptured aneurysm require immediate operation. Elective surgical or endovascular aortic repair (EVAR) is advisable for aneurysms that are large, i.e., > 5.5 cm (AAA or ascending TAA), or > 6 cm (descending TAA), symptomatic, or are growing rapidly. Patients with smaller aneurysms can be managed conservatively (risk factor modification, BP control, beta blockade) and followed by abdominal ultrasound (US) or CT scan every 6 to 12 months. Ultrasound screening for AAA is recommended for men age 65 to 75 who have smoked, and for those > 60 years with a family history of AAA.

Peripheral Arterial Disease

Peripheral arterial disease (PAD) generally refers to atherosclerotic occlusive disease in the arteries of the lower extremities. Mild PAD may be asymptomatic or cause intermittent claudication, a cramping pain in the legs induced by exercise and relieved by rest.

Treatment of PAD includes risk factor modification, exercise, and antiplatelet therapy (aspirin, clopidogrel, vorapaxar). Cilostazol (Pletal), a phosphodiesterase inhibitor-vasodilator with platelet inhibiting properties, has been shown to relieve symptoms and improve walking distance, and is recommended (if no CHF) in patients with intermittent claudication. Severe PAD usually requires percutaneous or surgical intervention, and as a last resort, amputation if critical limb ischemia is present. The prognosis for lower extremity PAD itself is generally good, although the mortality rate remains high because CAD and cerebrovascular disease often coexist.

Chapter 26. Pulmonary Hypertension

Pulmonary hypertension is defined as a hemodynamic state in which there is an elevation in mean pulmonary artery pressure of ≥ 25 mmHg at rest. Pulmonary artery pressure may increase secondary to:

- Progressive obliteration of small pulmonary arteries and arterioles (i.e., idiopathic or primary)
- An increase in pulmonary venous (left atrial) pressure caused by mitral valve disease or left heart failure (most common)
- Pulmonary parenchymal disease (hypoxemia)
- A reduction in the cross-sectional area of the pulmonary vascular bed (e.g., multiple pulmonary emboli)
- Miscellaneous disorders (multifactorial mechanisms)

Pulmonary hypertension can be classified into one of five types: *arterial, venous, hypoxic, thromboembolic, or miscellaneous*. This chapter will focus on the pharmacologic management of the patient who presents with idiopathic or primary pulmonary arterial hypertension.

Management of Pulmonary Arterial Hypertension

Treatment is rapidly evolving. Therapy may include:

- Cautious use of *vasodilators* (oral calcium channel blockers [in pulmonary vasodilator responders]) or continuous IV infusion of the vasodilator prostacyclin may relieve the pressure in the pulmonary circulation and benefit some patients. Prostacyclin analogs or other vasodilators, e.g., endothelin antagonists, or phosphodiesterase-5 inhibitors may be considered (in non-responders).
- Chronic *anticoagulation* therapy with warfarin (for in situ pulmonary thrombi) may also increase life expectancy.
- Portable *oxygen* (for marked hypoxemia at rest or during exercise testing) to maintain O_2 saturation at >90–92% (reduces hypoxic vasoconstriction).
- *Diuretics* for those with clinical signs of right-sided venous hypertension (elevated JVP, ascites, edema). Cautious diuresis since RV is preload dependent.

- *Digoxin*, often administered empirically, may counteract the potential negative inotropic effects of calcium channel blockers. Dobutamine can be used short term for decompensated pulmonary hypertension.
- *Balloon atrial septostomy* (R → L shunt causes ↑cardiac output, ↓ arterial oxygen saturation, net ↑tissue oxygen delivery).
- *Lung transplant* if the disease progresses despite maximal therapy. Heart-lung transplant needed if Eisenmenger physiology.

Vasodilator therapy particularly applies to those who respond favorably to a vasodilator challenge (e.g., IV prostacyclin, IV adenosine, inhaled nitric oxide) during right heart catheterization. Complications of pulmonary vasodilator therapy include systemic hypotension, hypoxemia, and even death. The most effective vasodilator is IV prostacyclin (epoprostenol [Flolan]), which is also the most complicated to administer (requires continuous infusion via a permanent venous catheter using a portable IV pump). This agent has been shown to decrease symptoms, increase exercise capacity, and decrease mortality in patients with idiopathic (primary) pulmonary hypertension. Current therapies for pulmonary arterial hypertension include vasoactive agents e.g., prostacyclin analogues (e.g., SQ, inhaled treprostinil [Remodulin, Tyvaso], inhaled iloprost [Ventavis]), endothelin-receptor antagonists (e.g., oral bosentan [Tracleer], oral ambrisentan [Letairis] oral macitentan [Opsumit]), phosphodiesterase-5 inhibitors (e.g., oral sildenafil [Revatio], oral tadalafil [Adcirca]), soluble guanylate cyclase stimulators (e.g., oral riociguat [Adempas]), and prostacyclin receptor agonists (e.g., oral selexipag [Uptravi]) which decreases pulmonary vascular resistance.

Overall, the outlook for patients with untreated idiopathic (primary) pulmonary hypertension remains poor (median survival 2.8 years). The prognosis is markedly improved if the patient responds to vasodilator therapy (up to 95% survival at 5 years). The outlook for patients with secondary pulmonary hypertension depends on the course of the underlying disease. The prognosis is generally favorable when pulmonary hypertension is detected early and the underlying cardiac and/or pulmonary diseases leading to it are treated appropriately.

Death in pulmonary arterial hypertension is most commonly due to right heart failure. In advanced stages, pulmonary artery pressures decline as the RV fails to generate enough blood flow to maintain high pressure. In select patients with advanced, refractory pulmonary hypertension, percutaneous balloon atrial septostomy may be considered as a bridge to lung transplantation or as a palliative treatment option. Creation of an intraatrial right-to-left shunt decompresses the failing right ventricle, increases LV filling, and improves cardiac output. Despite the decrease in arterial oxygen saturation that results, there is a net increase in tissue oxygen delivery. Improvement in survival and quality of life have been reported, but the procedure related mortality remains high. Lung transplantation should be considered if recurrent syncope and/or severe RV failure, refractory to medical therapy, are present. The 5 year survival rate following lung transplantation is ~45–55%.

Chapter 27.   Pericardial Disease

Diseases of the pericardium can produce a variety of clinical findings that may mimic many other organ system diseases e.g., pulmonary or liver disease, and be mistaken for other cardiac diagnoses, e.g., acute myocardial ischemia or infarction and chronic CHF. In this modern era of reperfusion therapy and aggressive intervention for acute coronary syndromes, investigation into such conditions as pericardial disease that are at especially high risk for developing hemorrhagic complications if inadvertently treated with thrombolytic agents and/or anticoagulant drugs is of the utmost importance. This chapter will highlight the clinical management of the common manifestations of pericardial heart disease.

Acute Pericarditis

Pericarditis is an inflammation of the visceral and/or parietal pericardium. It has numerous etiologies and the natural history depends to a great extent on the specific cause.

The most common cause is idiopathic, although the majority of these cases are likely due to viruses (e.g., Coxsackie A or B virus, influenza, HIV). Pericarditis may also result from an underlying malignancy (especially lung, breast, lymphoma), non-penetrating (e.g., steering wheel) chest injury, connective tissue disease (e.g., systemic lupus erythematosus, rheumatoid arthritis), certain medications (e.g., hydralazine, procainamide), and end-stage renal disease (uremic pericarditis). Pericarditis may also arise after an acute MI (early-contiguous, or late [10–14 days, *Dressler's syndrome*]), or cardiac injury (*post-pericardiotomy syndrome*).

The vast majority of cases of pericarditis are self-limited and uncomplicated. About 15–30% experience recurrences. The pain and inflammation is usually relieved by antiinflammatory agents, e.g., aspirin or NSAIDs (e.g., ibuprofen, indomethacin), with or without colchicine (to reduce recurrence). Steroids are not used routinely (because of their significant side effects) but may be reserved for uncontrolled pericarditis. Although they provide rapid and effective relief, steroids must be used cautiously, since an increased risk of recurrent pericarditis may develop when drug therapy is discontinued. Anticoagulation is not recommended due to the increased risk of pericardial hemorrhage and tamponade.

Cardiac Tamponade

In pericardial tamponade, fluid accumulates in the pericardial space, compresses the heart, and impairs diastolic filling and cardiac function. In *"slow tamponade"*, the patient may not appear acutely ill.

Conversely, in sudden massive tamponade, patients have rapid deterioration, and precipitous hypotension and death may occur. Cardiac tamponade is often rapid in onset and is frequently related to chest trauma (blunt or penetrating), infectious, uremic, or neoplastic disease. It may also occur during the first few days following cardiac surgery (intrapericardial bleeding). The degree of tamponade and hemodynamic embarrassment is related to the rapidity of fluid accumulation, not the quantity of fluid. Acute tamponade may occur with small pericardial effusions (even small amounts of fluid may cause significant elevation of pressure if the pericardium is noncompliant and stiff).

Urgent treatment by draining the pericardial fluid by needle (pericardiocentesis), or surgery (creating a pericardial window) is required to relieve cardiac compression. Removal of a small amount of fluid can be lifesaving.

Constrictive Pericarditis

Constrictive pericarditis is characterized by a thick, rigid, scarred, pericardium that restricts filling of all four chambers of the heart. It is usually a chronic consequence of acute or viral pericarditis, but may occur with carcinoma (especially breast and bronchogenic), prior radiation therapy to the chest for malignancy, and particularly following previous cardiac surgery.

Acute treatment usually includes gentle diuresis, whereas definitive therapy is surgical stripping of the pericardium.

Chapter 28.   Acute Cardiac Emergencies

The approach to the patient with an acute cardiac emergency requires astute evaluation and immediate intervention. This chapter will review the evaluation and treatment of the patient who presents with a sudden cardiac arrest, with a special emphasis on the basic and advanced cardiac life support measures used to preserve myocardial and cerebral viability, and treat potentially life threatening cardiac arrhythmias and shock.

General Considerations

Sudden cardiac death is generally defined as unexpected natural death from cardiac causes which occurs within one hour of the patient's collapse. Although sudden cardiac death may complicate a variety of cardiovascular diseases (e.g., HOCM; severe AS; dilated cardiomyopathy; MVP; prolonged QT, preexcitation [WPW], and Brugada's syndromes), coronary artery disease (with or without an acute MI) is by far the most common predisposing condition in patients with cardiac arrest. Regardless of the underlying etiology, cardiac arrest invariably results from one of the following rhythms:

- Ventricular fibrillation (VF)
- Pulseless ventricular tachycardia (VT)
- Pulseless electrical activity (PEA)
- Ventricular standstill (asystole)

The sudden collapse of an individual must be considered a cardiac arrest until proven otherwise. The approach to the patient involves the prompt and accurate recognition of a cardiac arrest, activation of the emergency response system (911 for out-of-hospital or "code blue" for in-hospital cardiac arrest), and rapid initiation of basic life support (BLS). The American Heart Association has issued updated guidelines on cardiopulmonary resuscitation (CPR) and emergency cardiac care. According to the guidelines, the BLS sequence of steps for trained rescuers has been changed from "**A-B-C**" (Airway, Breathing, Compressions) to "**C-A-B**" (Compressions, Airway, Breathing), to reflect our understanding of the positive impact on survival of early initiation of chest compressions, along with rapid Defibrillation (if pulseless VT and/or VF is present), often available via the use of automated external defibrillators (AEDs).

The key points to remember are the following:

- Cardiopulmonary resuscitation (CPR) comprises a series of steps aimed at the delivery of oxygenated blood to the heart and brain until spontaneous and effective circulation can be restored.

- Speed of diagnosis is critical. The chance of resuscitation diminishes (by ~ 7-10%) with each minute that has elapsed. Within 4 minutes of cardiac arrest, some cerebral damage is likely.

- Continuous chest compressions without assisted ventilation, i.e., cardiocerebral resuscitation (also known as "compression-only" or "hands-only" CPR) is an effective bystander approach to witnessed out-of-hospital cardiac arrest.

- A cardiac output of one fourth to one third can be achieved through external cardiac compression. Even these flow rates maintain adequate perfusion to the brain and other vital organs, thus preventing irreversible damage.

- Treat the *patient*, not the monitor.

- In patients with tachycardia or bradycardia who are hemodynamically stable, a 12 lead ECG can be helpful in making an accurate rhythm diagnosis and in guiding decisions regarding subsequent therapy.

- In patients with tachycardia who are hemodynamically unstable (manifested by hypotension, CHF, decreased level of consciousness, persistent chest pain), the decision to treat may need to be based on the presence or absence of heart sounds and/or pulses, or a single lead rhythm strip. In such cases, it is appropriate to treat a wide complex tachycardia as ventricular tachycardia until proven otherwise.

- The keys to the successful management of pulseless VT/VF are high quality CPR and early defibrillation (**Figure 28-1**).

- VF can usually be converted into a more stable rhythm when defibrillation occurs within the first few minutes (the "electrical phase"). Defibrillation alone (without chest compressions) is rarely successful when initiated after 4–5 minutes (the "circulatory phase").

- Defibrillator attempts should be preceded and followed by minimal interruptions in chest compressions.

- Survival rates for cardiac arrest are higher if the initial rhythm is "shockable" (pulseless VT/VF), the VF is "coarse", the arrest is "witnessed", and if it occurs "in-hospital" (especially in a monitored unit).

- The outcome from asystole and PEA is extremely poor despite treatment, with the exception of bradycardia due to hypoxemia from airway obstruction, hyperkalemia, drug overdose (e.g., digoxin, β-blocker, calcium channel blocker) or tamponade. Therefore, look for these reversible causes.

Figure 28-1

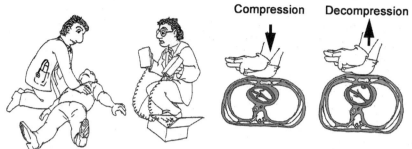

CARDIOPULMONARY RESUSCITATION (CPR)

Compression   Decompression

KEYS TO HIGH QUALITY CPR

- Push hard: 2-2.4 inches deep
- Push fast: 100-120 compressions/min
- Allow chest wall to completely recoil
- Minimize interruptions in chest compressions
- 30 compressions: 2 ventilations = 1 cycle of CPR
- Recheck pulse/rhythm and rotate compressors every 5 cycles (approx. 2 min) of CPR

- Early defibrillation (1 shock, not 3) for VF/pulseless VT
- Witnessed cardiac arrest: begin CPR, defibrillate x 1 ASAP, immediately resume CPR
- Unwitnessed cardiac arrest: CPR for 2 min ("prime the pump") first, then defibrillate x 1, and immediately resume CPR
- Consider early termination of resuscitation efforts for agonal rhythm and asystole

Note: High quality CPR and prompt defibrillation, when appropriate, are the only proven therapies to increase survival from cardiac arrest.

- After resuscitation of cardiac arrest, check for one of the following:
  —Reactive pupils, spontaneous respirations, and purposeful response to painful stimuli (signs associated with a high percentage of neurologic recovery).
  —Bilaterally dilated and fixed pupils (may be due to inadequate perfusion during cardiopulmonary resuscitation (CPR).
  —Unilateral pupil dilatation and unresponsiveness (which indicate a catastrophic central nervous system event and a dismal prognosis).
- Once a victim of cardiac arrest has been successfully resuscitated, consideration should be given to therapeutic hypothermia. Targeted temperature management (32–36° C in adults) and avoidance of hyperthermia may improve neurological outcomes and survival, and should be considered, along with urgent cardiac catheterization and PCI (if appropriate) in patients who remain comatose after resuscitation from cardiac arrest.

Survivors of cardiac arrest are at high risk for a recurrent episode if not evaluated and treated properly. Important information may be gained from interviewing the patient and/or the patient's family. A history of angina pectoris or a prior

MI indicates that CAD is likely present. If the cardiac arrest is preceded by chest pain (either during exertion or at rest), this may indicate that acute myocardial ischemia or infarction is responsible for precipitating the malignant ventricular arrhythmia. A history of dyspnea on exertion in the weeks or months preceding the cardiac arrest suggests that dilated cardiomyopathy, HOCM, or valvular heart disease, e.g., AS, may be present. A family history of sudden death raises the suspicion of long QT syndrome, HOCM, and rarely MVP and WPW syndrome with extremely rapid ventricular rates conducted over the accessory pathway that may precipitate VF. A drug history is important to obtain. VT may occur as a complication of certain antiarrhythmic drugs (proarrhythmic effect with long QT interval and polymorphic VT ["torsades de pointes"]), and diuretic-induced hypokalemia and hypomagnesemia. A history of alcohol consumption may suggest alcohol-induced cardiomyopathy and acutely predispose the patient to VT.

If the patient has been taking medications (e.g., digitalis, aminophylline) which could potentially precipitate a malignant ventricular arrhythmia, the serum levels of these drugs should be obtained. At times, it may be appropriate to order a toxicology screen if a drug overdose is suspected.

An echo-Doppler is often of great value in elucidating chamber size and function, along with the nature and severity of the patient's underlying structural heart disease (e.g., LV aneurysm, dilated cardiomyopathy, HOCM, AS, MVP). Radionuclide studies may also be helpful in select patients. Cardiac MRI is particularly valuable if arrhythmogenic RV dysplasia/cardiomyopathy (ARVD/C) is suspected. In most patients, cardiac catheterization is indicated either to elucidate the severity of structural heart disease which has been found by clinical and noninvasive evaluation, or to rule out occult forms of structural heart disease (e.g., CAD, congenital coronary abnormality) in patients who are not found to have identifiable heart disease after clinical and noninvasive evaluation. Invasive electrophysiologic testing also plays an important role in the diagnostic evaluation and management of patients who survive cardiac arrest. Following cardiac catheterization and/or electrophysiologic testing, an ICD (with or without antiarrhythmic drug therapy), and/or PCI, or cardiac surgery (CABG, aneurysmectomy, or resection/ablation of arrhythmic foci) is often necessary.

The algorithms that follow provide an overview of the approach to the patient with potentially life threatening cardiac arrhythmias including VF, pulseless VT, PEA asystole (no electrical activity), bradycardia with pulses, tachycardia with pulses, as well as shock (**Figures 28-2 through 28-10**). The content of these protocols is based on the 2018 guidelines update on advanced cardiac life support (ACLS) established by the American Heart Association (AHA) and the Emergency Cardiac Care Committee.

Figures 28-2 through 28-10. Advanced Cardiac Life Support and Shock Algorithms. (Modified from Hancock, J. The Practitioner's Pocket Pal. MedMaster, Inc. 2012).

Figure 28-2

UNIVERSAL ALGORITHM

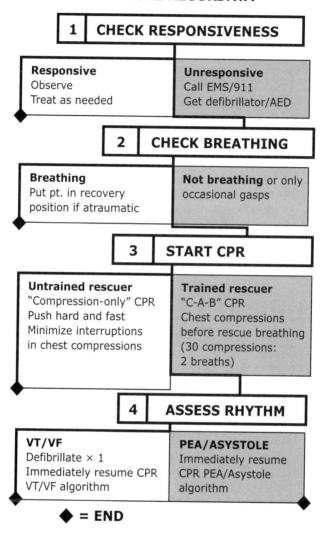

1	CHECK RESPONSIVENESS

Responsive Observe Treat as needed	**Unresponsive** Call EMS/911 Get defibrillator/AED

2	CHECK BREATHING

Breathing Put pt. in recovery position if atraumatic	**Not breathing** or only occasional gasps

3	START CPR

Untrained rescuer "Compression-only" CPR Push hard and fast Minimize interruptions in chest compressions	**Trained rescuer** "C-A-B" CPR Chest compressions before rescue breathing (30 compressions: 2 breaths)

4	ASSESS RHYTHM

VT/VF Defibrillate × 1 Immediately resume CPR VT/VF algorithm	**PEA/ASYSTOLE** Immediately resume CPR PEA/Asystole algorithm

◆ = END

Note: EMS: Emergency Medical Services; AED: Automated External Defibrillator; CPR: Cardiopulmonary Resuscitation; C-A-B: Compressions, Airway, Breathing; VT/VF: pulseless Ventricular Tachycardia/Ventricular Fibrillation; PEA: Pulseless Electrical Activity.

Figure 28-3

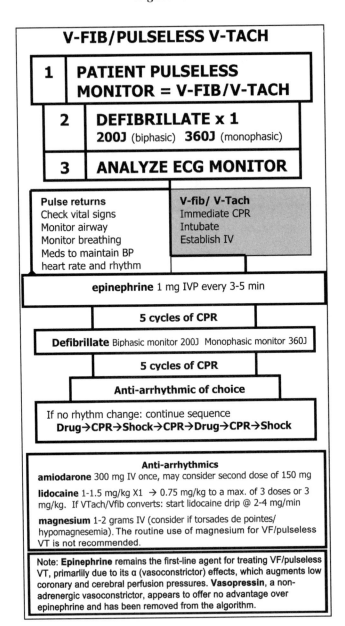

V-FIB/PULSELESS V-TACH

1	PATIENT PULSELESS MONITOR = V-FIB/V-TACH

2	**DEFIBRILLATE x 1** 200J (biphasic) **360J** (monophasic)

3	**ANALYZE ECG MONITOR**

Pulse returns
Check vital signs
Monitor airway
Monitor breathing
Meds to maintain BP
heart rate and rhythm

V-fib/ V-Tach
Immediate CPR
Intubate
Establish IV

epinephrine 1 mg IVP every 3-5 min

5 cycles of CPR

Defibrillate Biphasic monitor 200J Monophasic monitor 360J

5 cycles of CPR

Anti-arrhythmic of choice

If no rhythm change: continue sequence
Drug→CPR→Shock→CPR→Drug→CPR→Shock

Anti-arrhythmics
amiodarone 300 mg IV once, may consider second dose of 150 mg

lidocaine 1-1.5 mg/kg X1 → 0.75 mg/kg to a max. of 3 doses or 3 mg/kg. If VTach/Vfib converts: start lidocaine drip @ 2-4 mg/min

magnesium 1-2 grams IV (consider if torsades de pointes/ hypomagnesemia). The routine use of magnesium for VF/pulseless VT is not recommended.

Note: **Epinephrine** remains the first-line agent for treating VF/pulseless VT, primarlily due to its α (vasoconstrictor) effects, which augments low coronary and cerebral perfusion pressures. **Vasopressin**, a non-adrenergic vasoconstrictor, appears to offer no advantage over epinephrine and has been removed from the algorithm.

Figure 28-4

PULSELESS ELECTRICAL ACTIVITY

1	ECG SHOWS PEA
2	CPR → INTUBATE ESTABLISH IV
3	CONSIDER POSSIBLE CAUSE & TREAT

Cause*	Treatment
1. Hypovolemia	1. Fluid challenge
2. Cardiac tamponade	2. Pericardiocentesis
3. Hypoxia	3. Airway/ventilation
4. Acidosis	4. $NaHCO_3$ (1meq/kg)
5. Tension pneumothorax	5. Chest decompression
6. Hypothermia	6. Rewarming
7. Pulmonary embolism	7. Thrombolytics** or surgery
8. Drug overdose	8. Treat per drug
9. Hyperkalemia	9. $CaCl_2$ 1 amp IV over 5 min.→ reg. insulin 5 units IV with 50 cc D50W. → $NaHCO_3$ 1meq/kg
10. MI	10. See MI protocol

epinephrine 1 mg IVP every 3-5 minutes
(may give as soon as feasible after cardiac arrest due to nonshockable rhythm)

Heart Rate < 60	Heart Rate > 60
Atropine 1 mg IVP every 3-5 min (up to 3 doses)***	Continue with epinephrine

Note: * When considering the causes of pulseless electrical activity (PEA) or asystole, keep in mind the 5 "H's" and 5 "T's": **H**ypovolemia, **H**ypoxia, **H**ydrogen ion (acidosis), **H**yperkalemia, **H**ypothermia, and **T**ablets/**T**oxins (drug overdose), **T**amponade (cardiac), **T**ension pneumothorax, **T**hrombosis, coronary (MI), and **T**hromboembolism, pulmonary. ** Thrombolysis following *aggressive* CPR may cause cardiac tamponade. *** Atropine is unlikely to have a therapeutic benefit and is no longer recommended for routine use in PEA or asystole.

Figure 28-5

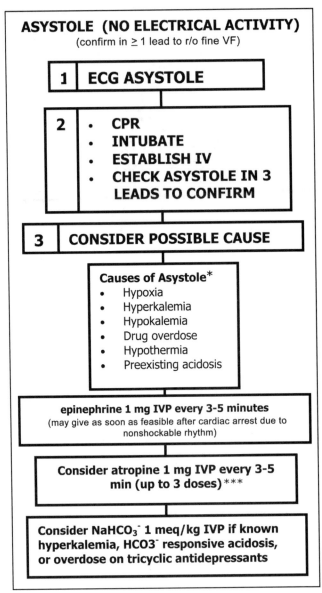

ASYSTOLE (NO ELECTRICAL ACTIVITY)
(confirm in ≥ 1 lead to r/o fine VF)

1 | ECG ASYSTOLE

2 |
- **CPR**
- **INTUBATE**
- **ESTABLISH IV**
- **CHECK ASYSTOLE IN 3 LEADS TO CONFIRM**

3 | CONSIDER POSSIBLE CAUSE

Causes of Asystole*
- Hypoxia
- Hyperkalemia
- Hypokalemia
- Drug overdose
- Hypothermia
- Preexisting acidosis

epinephrine 1 mg IVP every 3-5 minutes
(may give as soon as feasible after cardiac arrest due to nonshockable rhythm)

Consider atropine 1 mg IVP every 3-5 min (up to 3 doses) *

Consider NaHCO$_3^-$ 1 meq/kg IVP if known hyperkalemia, HCO3$^-$ responsive acidosis, or overdose on tricyclic antidepressants

Note: * When considering the causes of pulseless electrical activity (PEA) or asystole, keep in mind the 5 "H's" and 5 "T's": Hypovolemia, Hypoxia, Hydrogen ion (acidosis), Hyperkalemia, Hypothermia, and Tablets/Toxins (drug overdose), Tamponade (cardiac), Tension pneumothorax, Thrombosis, coronary (MI), and Thromboembolism, pulmonary. ** Thrombolysis following *aggressive* CPR may cause cardiac tamponade. *** Atropine is unlikely to have a therapeutic benefit and is no longer recommended for routine use in PEA or asystole.

Figure 28-6

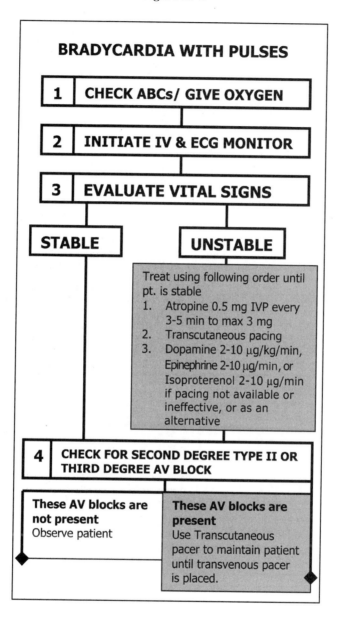

Figure 28-7

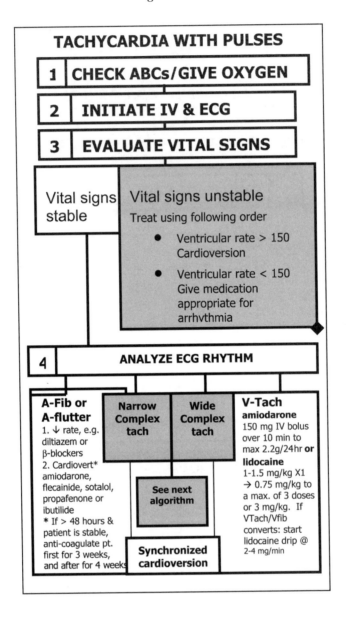

Figure 28-8

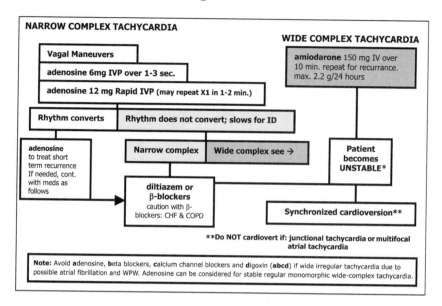

*Note: When evaluating if a patient is unstable, keep in mind the mnemonic **"CASH"**: **C**hest pain, **A**ltered mental status, **S**hortness of breath, and **H**ypotension. (You don't get the 'joules' if you don't have the 'CASH'!)

Figure 28-9

SHOCK

Definition: Inadequate perfusion resulting in poor oxygenation of body tissues, which can cause cellular and organ damage.

Signs & Symptoms: All types of shock share the above definition and therefore share a set of common signs and symptoms which may result from insufficient perfusion of the following organ systems.

- Central nervous system
  - Confusion
  - Anxiety
  - Belligerence or agitation
  - Decreased level of consciousness
  - Loss of consciousness
  - Coma
- Circulatory system
  - Weak pulses
  - Tachycardia
  - Hypotension
  - Edema (Anaphylactic & Septic)
- Integument
  - Peripheral cyanosis
  - Mottling
  - Slow capillary refill
  - Cool extremities
  - Flushing (Septic & Anaphylactic)
- Renal
  - Decreased urine output
  - May present in pre renal failure

Types of Shock:
- HYPOVOLEMIC
  - Loss of intravascular volume due to blood loss, third spacing of fluid or dehydration
- CARDIOGENIC
  - Inability to properly circulate blood volume due to cardiac pump failure
- ANAPHYLACTIC
  - Inability to perfuse due to massive third spacing of fluid resulting in intravascular hypovolemia
  - Inability to oxygenate blood due to bronchial edema and secretion
- SEPTIC
  - Inability to perfuse due to third spacing of fluids and or infection of vital organ systems
- NEUROGENIC
  - Inability to perfuse due to generalized vasodilation and subsequent loss of blood pressure resulting from loss of autonomic vascular tone

Figure 28-10

TREATMENT OF SHOCK

1	**ASSESS ABCs & LOC**

2	**ESTABLISH IV ACCESS**

3	**DETERMINE CAUSE OF SHOCK**

4	TREAT ACCORDINGLY

HYPOVOLEMIC:
1. Place patient in Trendelenburg position
2. Fluid challenge with Normal Saline, Lactated Ringer's or blood transfusion, and continuously reassess vital signs
3. Find and treat cause of volume loss

CARDIOGENIC:
1. Fluid bolus 250 cc at a time with continuous reassessment of vital signs and lung sounds for pulmonary edema*
2. Consider inotropic drugs e.g.
   - Dopamine 2.5-20 μg/kg/min IV
   - Dobutamine 2-20 μg/kg/min IV
   - Norepinephrine 0.5-30 μg/min IV

ANAPHYLACTIC:
1. Support airway, may require intubation; O2
2. Fluid challenge with Normal Saline or Lactated Ringers
3. Epinephrine 0.3 mg 1:1000 SC
4. Diphenhydramine 50 mg IV

SEPTIC:
1. Fluid bolus 250 cc at a time with continuous reassessment of vital signs and lung sounds for pulmonary edema
2. Find site of infection and treat

NEUROGENIC (VASODILATION):
1. If cause is unknown, consider traumatic and protect cervical spine and properly immobilize patient
2. Fluid bolus 250 cc at a time with continuous reassessment of vital signs and lung sounds for pulmonary edema
3. Find cause and treat accordingly

IF PULMONARY EDEMA WITH CARDIOGENIC SHOCK:

First-line actions	Also consider
Lasix IV 0.5-1.0 mg/kg	Nitroglycerin IV for BP>100 mmHg
Morphine IV 1-3 mg	Nitroprusside IV for BP>100 mmHg
Nitroglycerin SL	Dopamine for BP<100 mmHg
Oxygen/intubate PRN	Dobutamine for BP<100 mmHg
	IABP, eval. need for PCI/surgery

171

Appendix. Cardiac Drug Dosages And Indications

Below is a table of common cardiac drugs, along with drug classes, alphabetized by both generic and brand names. While current drug dosages and indications are provided, it remains the responsibility of today's practitioner to evaluate the appropriateness of therapy and dosing in the context of the clinical situation of an individual patient. Because standards for usage periodically change, it is advisable to keep abreast of revised recommendations, particularly regarding new or infrequently used drugs.

COMMON CARDIAC DRUGS		
Drug	**Dose**	**Comments**
I. β-Blockers ("-olols") β-Blockers are not first line agents for HTN (unless angina, MI, or heart failure is present). Contraindicated with acute decompensated heart failure, cardiogenic shock, heart block greater than first degree, severe bradycardia, or sick sinus syndrome (without pacemaker). Agents with intrinsic sympathomimetic activity (e.g., pindolol) are contraindicated post-MI. Abrupt cessation may precipitate angina, MI, arrhythmias, tachycardia, rebound HTN. Patients currently taking cocaine should avoid β-blockers with unopposed α-adrenergic vasoconstriction since this will promote coronary spasm (carvedilol or labetalol have α-1-blocking effects and may be safer). Concomitant amiodarone, disopyramide, clonidine, digoxin, or nondihydropyridine calcium channel blockers may increase risk of bradycardia. Monitor for heart failure exacerbation and hypotension (particularly orthostatic) when titrating dose. All β-blockers, except carvedilol, may increase blood glucose or mask tachycardia occurring with hypoglycemia. May aggravate symptoms of PAD. Non-selective β-blockers, including carvedilol and labetalol, are contraindicated with asthma.		
Acebutolol (Sectral)	**HTN**: Start 400 mg PO daily or 200 mg PO twice daily, max 1200 mg/day.	Cardioselective (β-1); has mild intrinsic sympathomimetic activity.
Atenolol (Tenormin)	**Acute MI**: 50-100 mg PO daily or in divided doses; or 5 mg IV over 5 min followed by another 5 mg injection 10 min later. **HTN**: Start 25-50 mg PO daily or divided twice daily, max 100 mg/day.	Cardioselective (β-1). May be less effective for HTN and lowering CV event risk than other β-blockers.
Bisoprolol (Zebeta)	**HTN**: Start 2.5 - 5 mg PO daily, max 20 mg/day. **Heart failure with reduced ejection fraction**: Start 1.25 mg PO daily, max 10mg/day	Highly Cardioselective (β-1).

Carvedilol (Coreg, Coreg CR)	**Heart failure**: Immediate-release: Start 3.125 mg PO twice daily, double dose q 2 weeks up to max of 25 mg twice daily (for wt ≤ 85 kg) or 50 mg twice daily (for wt > 85 kg). **Sustained-release**: Start 10 mg PO daily, double dose q 2 weeks as tolerated up to max of 80 mg/day. **LV dysfunction following acute MI**: Immediate-release: Start 3.125 - 6.25 mg PO twice daily, double dose q 3 - 10 days as tolerated to max of 25 mg twice daily. Sustained-release: Start 10 - 20 mg PO daily, double dose q 3 - 10 days as tolerated; max 80 mg/day. **HTN**: Immediate-release: Start 6.25 mg PO twice daily, double dose q 7 - 14 days as tolerated to max 50 mg/day. Sustained-release: Start 20 mg PO daily, double dose q 7 -14 days as tolerated to max 80 mg/day.	Combined α-1, β-1, and β-2 receptor blocker.
Esmolol (Brevibloc)	**SVT/HTN emergency**: Load 500 mcg/kg over 1 min, then start infusion 50 to 200 mcg/kg/min	β-1 receptor selective. Half-life is 9 min.
Labetalol (Trandate)	**HTN**: Start 100 mg PO twice daily, max 2400 mg/day. **HTN emergency**: Start 20 mg IV slow injection, then 40 - 80 mg IV q 10 min prn up to 300 mg or IV infusion 0.5 - 2 mg/min.	Combined α-1, β-1, and β-2 receptor blocker. May be used to manage HTN during pregnancy.
Metoprolol Succinate (Toprol-XL)	**HTN**: Start 25 - 100 mg PO daily, may double dose q week, max 400 mg/day. **Heart failure**: Start 12.5 - 25 mg PO daily, may double dose q 2 weeks, max 200 mg/day. **Angina**: Start 100 mg PO daily, may double dose q week, max 400 mg/day.	Cardioselective (β-1). Metoprolol succinate is extended-release form.

COMMON CARDIAC DRUGS (*Continued*)		
Drug	**Dose**	**Comments**
Metoprolol Tartrate (Lopressor)	**HTN**: Start 100 mg PO daily or in divided doses, max 450 mg/day. **Angina**: Start 50 mg PO twice daily, max 400 mg/day. **Acute MI**: Give 5 mg IV-bolus every 2 min for 3 doses based on BP, HR, and ECG response; wait 15 min, then 25 - 50 mg PO q 6 h for 48 h; then 100 mg PO q 12 h.	Cardioselective (β-1). Metoprolol tartrate is immediate-release form.
Nadolol (Corgard)	**HTN**: Start 20 - 40 mg PO daily, max 320 mg/day.	Noncardioselective (β-1 & β-2).
Nebivolol (Bystolic)	**HTN**: Start 5 mg PO daily, max 40 mg/day.	Dose $\leq$ 10 mg or extensive metabolizer: β-1 selective. Dose > 10 mg or poor metabolizer: β-1 & β-2 blocker. Vasodilatory properties.
Pindolol (Visken)	**HTN**: Start 5 mg PO twice daily, max 60 mg/day.	β-1 & β-2 receptor blocker. Intrinsic sympathomimetic activity.
Propranolol (Inderal, Inderal LA)	**HTN**: Start 20 - 40 mg PO twice daily or 60 - 80 mg PO daily, max 640 mg/day; extended-release (Inderal LA) max 640 mg/day. **SVT or rapid atrial fibrillation/ flutter**: 1 mg IV q 2 min, max 2 doses in 4 h.	β-1 & β-2 receptor blocker.
Timolol (Blocadren)	**HTN**: Start 10 mg PO twice daily, max 60 mg/day.	β-1 & β-2 receptor blocker.

II. Nitrates

Avoid if systolic BP < 90 mmHg, severe bradycardia, tachycardia, severe AS, or RV infarction (preload sensitive). Avoid if patient takes PDE-5 inhibitors (e.g. Sildenafil, Tadalafil, Vardenafil) or soluble guanylate cyclase stimulators (e.g. Riociguat).

Isosorbide dinitrate (Isordil, Dilatrate-SR)	**Angina prophylaxis**: 5 - 40 mg PO three times daily (7 am, noon, 5 pm), sustained-release: 40 - 80 mg PO twice daily (8 am, 2 pm).	
Isosorbide mononitrate (Imdur, Ismo)	**Angina**: 20 mg PO twice daily (8 am and 3 pm). Extended-release: Start 30 - 60 mg PO daily, max 240 mg/day.	Do not use for acute angina.
Nitroglycerin IV	**Perioperative HTN, acute MI, heart failure, acute angina**: Start 5 - 10 mcg/min, titrate by 10 mcg/min every 3-5 min prn.	
Nitroglycerin ointment (Nitro-BID)	**Angina prophylaxis**: Start 0.5 inches q 8 h, maintenance 1 - 2 inches q 8 h, max 4 inches q 4 - 6 h.	Allow for a nitrate-free period of 10 - 14 h to avoid nitrate tolerance. Do not use for acute angina.
Nitroglycerin spray (Nitrolingual, NitroMist)	**Acute angina**: 1 - 2 sprays under the tongue prn, max 3 sprays in 15 min.	
Nitroglycerin sublingual (Nitrostat)	**Acute angina, sublingual tabs**: 0.4 mg SL, repeat dose q 5 min prn up to 3 doses in 15 min. **Acute angina, sublingual powder**: 0.4 - 0.8 mg SL, repeat dose q 5 min prn up to 1.2 mg total in 15 min.	
Nitroglycerin sustained release	**Angina prophylaxis**: Start 2.5 mg PO twice daily, then titrate upward prn.	
Nitroglycerin transdermal (Minitran, Nitro-Dur)	**Angina prophylaxis**: 1 patch 12 - 14 h each day.	Allow for a nitrate-free period of 10 - 14 h to avoid nitrate tolerance. Do not use for acute angina.

COMMON CARDIAC DRUGS (*Continued*)

Drug	Dose	Comments
IIa. Other Anti-anginal Agents		
Ranolazine (Ranexa)	**Chronic angina**: 500 mg PO twice daily, max 1000 mg twice daily. Limit dose to 500 mg twice daily if used with diltiazem or verapamil (which increases plasma level of ranolazine).	Prolongs QT interval. If CrCl <60 mL/min at baseline, monitor renal function; discontinue ranolazine if acute renal failure occurs. Avoid with long QT interval, QT prolonging drugs, or liver disease. Approved for use with nitrates, β-blockers, or amlodipine.
III. Dihydropyridine Calcium Channel Blockers ("-dipines") Avoid in decompensated heart failure. May increase peripheral edema. Avoid grapefruit juice.		
Amlodipine (Norvasc)	**HTN**: Start 5 mg PO daily, max 10 mg/day. Elderly, small, frail, or with liver disease: Start 2.5 PO daily.	
Clevidipine (Cleviprex)	**HTN**: Start 1-2 mg/h IV, titrate q 1.5 - 10 min to BP response, usual maintenance dose 4 - 6 mg/h, max 32 mg/h IV.	Used for hypertensive emergency
Felodipine (Plendil)	**HTN**: Start 2.5 - 5 mg PO daily, max 10 mg/day.	
Isradipine (Dynacirc CR)	**HTN**: Start 2.5 mg PO twice daily, max 20 mg/day (max 10 mg/day in elderly).	
Nicardipine (Cardene)	**HTN**: Start IV infusion at 5 mg/h, titrate to effect, max 15 mg/h. **HTN**: Start 20 mg PO three times daily, max 120 mg/day.	Used for hypertensive emergency.

Nifedipine (Procardia, Adalat, Procardia XL, Adalat CC, Afeditab CR, Adalat XL)	HTN/angina: Extended-release: 30 - 60 mg PO daily, max 120 mg/day. Angina: Immediate-release: Start 10 mg PO three times daily, max 120 mg/day.	Avoid sublingual use, may cause excessive hypotension, acute MI, CVA. Do not use immediate-release form for treating HTN, hypertensive emergencies, or ST-elevation MI.

IV. Nondihydropyridine Calcium Channel Blockers
Avoid in decompensated heart failure, 2nd/3rd degree heart block without pacemaker, acute MI and pulmonary congestion, or systolic BP <90 mm Hg.

Diltiazem (Cardizem, Cardizem LA, Cardizem CD, Cartia XT, Dilacor XR, Diltiazem CD, Taztia XT, Tiazac)	**Atrial fibrillation/flutter, PSVT**: IV Bolus 20 mg (0.25 mg/kg) over 2 min. Re-bolus 15 min later (if needed) 25 mg (0.35 mg/kg). Infusion 5-15 mg/h. **HTN, once daily, extended-release**: Start 120-240 mg PO daily, max 540 mg/day. **HTN, twice daily, sustained release**: Start 60-120 mg PO twice daily, max 360 mg/day. **Angina, immediate-release**: Start 30 mg PO four times daily, max 360 mg/day divided three to four times daily. **Angina, extended-release**: Start 120-240 mg PO daily, max 540 mg/day.	
Verapamil (Isoptin SR, Calan, Calan SR, Verelan, Verelan PM)	**SVT**: 5 -10 mg IV over 2 min. **Angina:** Immediate-release: start 40 - 80 mg PO three to four times daily, max 480 mg/day. Sustained-release: Start 120 - 240 mg PO daily, max 480 mg/day (use twice daily dosing for doses > 240 mg/day with Isoptin SR and Calan SR). **HTN**: Same as angina, except (Verelan PM) 100 to 200 mg PO at bedtime, max 400 mg/day; immediate-release tabs should be avoided in treating HTN.	Use cautiously with impaired renal/hepatic function. May cause constipation.

COMMON CARDIAC DRUGS (*Continued*)		
Drug	**Dose**	**Comments**
V. Antiplatelet Agents		
Aspirin (acetylsalicylic acid, Ecotrin, Empirin, Half-prin, Bayer, Anacin)	**ACS**: 162 – 325 mg PO x 1 dose (non-enteric coated, chewable), then 81 mg PO daily. **CAD** (chronic therapy): 81-325 mg PO daily.	If allergy, use clopidogrel and/or desensitize to aspirin. Should not be stopped prior to CABG surgery.
Aggrenox (Aspirin + dipyridamole)	**Prevention of CVA after TIA/CVA**: 1 cap PO twice daily. **Ecotrin**	Headache is a common adverse effect.
Cilostazol (Pletal)	**Intermittent claudication**: 100 mg PO twice daily. 50 mg PO twice daily with CYP3A4 inhibitors (e.g., keto-conazole, itraconazole, erythromycin, dil-tiazem) or CYP2C19 inhibitors (e.g., omeprazole).	Contraindicated in heart failure due to decreased survival.
Cangrelor (Kengreal)	**Adjunct to PCI**: Load 30 mcg/kg IV prior to PCI, then IV infusion 4 mcg/kg/min for at least 2 h or until end of procedure, whichever is longer.	IV P2Y12 inhibitor. Rapid onset/offset. Adjunct to PCI to reduce thrombotic events, including peripro-cedural MI, repeat coronary revascularization, and stent thrombosis, in patients who have not been treated with P2Y12 inhibitor and GP IIb/IIIa inhibitor.
Clopidogrel (Plavix)	**Prior to or at time of PCI**: 300 - 600 mg PO x 1, then 75 mg PO daily. **ACS**: 300 - 600 mg loading dose, then 75 mg PO daily. **Recent acute MI/CVA, established PAD**: 75 mg PO daily without a loading dose.	D/C 5 days prior to CABG surgery. Concomitant morphine use may delay and reduce absorption of clopidogrel. Avoid drugs that are strong or moderate CYP2C19 in-hibitors (e.g., omeprazole, esomeprazole, cimetidine, fluconazole, fluoxetine, ketoconazole).

Prasugrel (Effient)	**ACS managed with PCI**: 60 mg x 1 at time of PCI, then 10 mg PO daily. If weight < 60 kg, consider 5 mg PO daily.	More rapid and potent platelet inhibitor than clopidogrel. Give at time of PCI and not upstream due to ↑ bleeding risk. D/C 7 days prior to CABG surgery. Concomitant morphine use may delay and reduce absorption of prasugrel. Contraindicated if history of TIA or CVA. Avoid if age ≥ 75 yrs. Risk factors for bleeding: wt <60 kg, concomitant meds that increase bleeding risk.
Ticagrelor (Brilinta)	**ACS or history of MI**: 180 mg PO x 1, then 90 mg PO twice daily x 1 year post-ACS, then 60 mg PO twice daily or may switch to clopidogrel.	More rapid and potent platelet inhibitor than clopidogrel. Give upstream or at time of PCI. D/C 5 days prior to CABG surgery. Concomitant morphine use may delay and reduce absorption of ticagrelor. Give with aspirin; after any initial dose, use with aspirin max 75 - 100 mg daily. Do not use with history of intracranial hemorrhage, active bleeding, or severe liver disease. May cause dyspnea and ventricular pauses (adenosine effect).
Vorapaxar (Zontivity)	**History of MI or PAD**: 2.08 mg PO daily.	Reduces thrombotic events in patients with history of MI or PAD. Do not use with active bleeding or history of TIA or CVA.

COMMON CARDIAC DRUGS (*Continued*)		
Drug	**Dose**	**Comments**
VI. Glycoprotein (GP) IIb/IIIa Antagonists No clear benefit for routinely starting prior to PCI and ↑bleeding risk. Consider if high risk ACS, especially if refractory ischemia, large clot burden at time of PCI, and/or inadequate pre-treatment with dual antiplatelet therapy.		
Abciximab (ReoPro)	**PCI**: 0.25 mg/kg IV bolus over 5 min given 10-60 min prior to PCI, then 0.125 mcg/kg/min (max 10 mcg/min) IV infusion for 12 h. **ACS (unresponsive to standard therapy when PCI is planned within 24 hr)**: 0.25 mg/kg IV bolus over 5 min, followed by a 10 mcg/min IV infusion for 18-24 hr prior to PCI and continued until 1 hr after PCI	Thrombocytopenia possible; monitor platelets.
Eptifibatide (Integrilin)	**ACS**: Load 180 mcg/kg IV bolus, then infuse 2 mcg/kg/min for up to 72 h. Discontinue prior to CABG surgery. **PCI**: Load 180 mcg/kg IV bolus just before procedure, followed by infusion of 2 mcg/kg/min and a 2nd 180 mcg/kg IV bolus 10 min after the first bolus. Continue infusion for up to 18 to 24 h (minimum 12 h) after procedure. CrCl <50 mL/min not on dialysis: Reduce infusion rate to 1 mcg/kg/min. Dialysis: contraindicated.	Thrombocytopenia possible; monitor platelets.
Tirofiban (Aggrastat)	**ACS**: Give 25 mcg/kg within 5 min, then 0.15 mcg/kg/min for up to 18 h. Renal impairment (CrCl ≤60 mL/min): Give 25 mcg/kg within 5 min, then 0.075 mcg/kg/min.	Thrombocytopenia possible; monitor platelets.

VIIa. Anticoagulants – Direct Thrombin Inhibitors

Bivalirudin (Angiomax)	**During PCI (with or without HIT/HITTS) or PTCA (without HIT/HITTS):** 0.75 mg/kg IV bolus prior to intervention, then 1.75 mg/kg/h until end of procedure. May continue infusion up to 4 h post-procedure (should be strongly considered post-STEMI to reduce risk of stent thrombosis), then may additionally infuse 0.2 mg/kg/h for up to 20 h more. For CrCl <30 mL/min, reduce infusion dose.	Use with aspirin 300 - 325 mg PO daily. Decreases bleeding risk (compared to unfractionated heparin and GP IIb/IIIa inhibitor). If HIT/HITTS, use bivalirudin instead of unfractionated heparin.
Dabigatran (Pradaxa)	**Stroke prevention in nonvalvular atrial fibrillation**: 150 mg PO twice daily; CrCl 15 - 30 mL/min: 75 mg PO twice daily; CrCl < 15 mL/min, contraindicated.	Contraindicated in mechanical prosthetic heart valves (use warfarin). Specific reversal agent available: Idarucizumab (Praxbind).

VIIb. Anticoagulants—Factor Xa Inhibitors ("-aban")

Apixaban (Eliquis)	**Stroke prevention in nonvalvular atrial fibrillation**: 5 mg PO twice daily. Reduce dose to 2.5 mg PO twice daily if ≥2 of the following characteristics: age ≥80 yr, wt ≤60 kg, serum Cr ≥1.5 mg/dL.	Contraindicated in mechanical prosthetic heart valves (use warfarin). Specific reversal agent available: Adnexanet alfa (Andexxa)
Edoxaban (Savaysa, Lixiana)	**Stroke prevention in nonvalvular atrial fibrillation**: CrCl 50 - 95 mL/min: 60 mg PO daily. CrCl 15 to 50 mL/min: 30 mg PO daily.	Contraindicated in mechanical prosthetic heart valves (use warfarin). Specific reversal agent available: Adnexanet (Andexxa)

COMMON CARDIAC DRUGS (*Continued*)		
Drug	**Dose**	**Comments**
Fondaparinux (Arixtra)	**ACS**: 2.5 mg SC daily	Increased risk of catheter thrombosis; supplement with unfractionated heparin if PCI.
Rivaroxaban (Xarelto)	**Stroke prevention in nonvalvular atrial fibrillation**: 20 mg PO daily with evening meal; if CrCl ≤50 mL/min, 15 mg PO daily with evening meal. **Reduction of risk of major cardiovascular events in chronic CAD or PAD**: 2.5 mg PO twice daily, with or without food, in combination with aspirin (75-100 mg) once daily.	Contraindicated in mechanical prosthetic heart valves (use warfarin). Specific reversal agent available: Adnexanet (Andexxa).
VIIc. Anticoagulants—Low Molecular Weight Heparins (LWMH)		
Enoxaparin (Lovenox)	**ACS**: 1 mg/kg SC q 12 h. If CrCl <30 mL/min, 1 mg/kg SC once daily. **STEMI in age <75 yr**: 30 mg IV bolus with 1 mg/kg SC dose, then 1 mg/kg SC q 12 h (max 100 mg/dose for the 1st two doses). If CrCl <30 mL/min, 30 mg IV bolus with 1 mg/kg SC dose, then 1 mg/kg SC daily. **STEMI in age ≥75 yr**: No IV bolus, 0.75 mg/kg SC q 12 h (max 75 mg/dose for the 1st two doses). If CrCl <30 mL/min, no IV bolus, 1 mg/kg SC daily.	

VIId. Anticoagulants—Other

Unfraction-ated Hepa-rin (UFH)	**STEMI**: With thrombolyt-ics: Bolus 60 IU/kg IV load (max 4000 IU), then initial infusion 12 IU/kg/h (max 1000 IU/h) adjusted to target aPTT 1.5 - 2 times control. **ACS with or without PCI**: Bolus 60 IU/kg IV (max 4000 IU), then 12 IU/kg/h (max 1000 IU/h) infusion, adjust to target aPTT 1.5 to 2 times control.	Monitor aPTT 6 h after heparin initiation and 6 h after each dosage adjustment. When aPTT is stable within therapeutic range, monitor daily. Thrombocytopenia possible; monitor platelets. May begin warfarin on 1 day of heparin; continue heparin for at least 4–5 days of combined therapy.
Warfarin (Coumadin, Jantoven)	For inpatient therapy, start 2 - 5 mg PO daily for 1 to 2 days, then adjust to target INR. For outpatient therapy, may start 10 mg PO daily for 2 days, then adjust to target INR. **Target 2.0–3.0**: A fib, DVT, PE, bioprosthetic mitral heart valve, mechanical prosthetic aortic heart valve. **Target 2.5–3.5**: Mechanical prosthetic heart valve (mitral position, aortic position with risk factors for thromboembolism*).	*Risk factors for thromboembolism: atrial fibrillation, previous thromboembolism, LV dysfunction, and hypercoagulable states.

VIII. Thrombolytics ("Clot busters")

Alteplase (tPA, Activase)	**Acute MI**: <u>wt 67 kg or less</u>, give 15 mg IV bolus, then 0.75 mg/kg (max 50 mg) over 30 min, then 0.5 mg/kg (max 35 mg) over the next 60 min; <u>wt greater than 67 kg</u>, give 15 mg IV bolus, then 50 mg over 30 min, then 35 mg over the next 60 min.	Absolute contraindications: previous intracerebral hemorrhage; intracranial neoplasm, aneurysm, AV malformation; recent (< 3 months) ischemic CVA (except acute ischemic CVA < 4.5 hours); active bleeding or bleeding diathesis (excluding menses); significant closed head or facial trauma (< 3 months); suspected aortic dissection.

COMMON CARDIAC DRUGS (*Continued*)

Drug	Dose	Comments
Anistreplase (Eminase)	**STEMI**: 30 IU IV over 2-5 min.	
Reteplase (rPA)	**STEMI**: 10 units IV over 2 min, repeat x 1 dose in 30 min.	
Streptokinase (Kabikinase, Streptase)	**STEMI**: 1.5 MU IV over 60 min.	Contraindicated in prior streptokinase exposure.
Tenecteplase (TNKase)	**STEMI**: Single IV bolus dose over 5 sec based on weight: wt < 60 kg: 30 mg; wt 60 - 69 kg: 35 mg; wt 70 - 79 kg: 40 mg; wt 80 - 89 kg: 45 mg; wt ≥ 90 kg: 50 mg.	
IX. Cardiac Glycosides		
Digoxin (Lanoxin, Digitek)	**Systolic heart failure, rate control of chronic atrial fibrillation**: Age <70 yrs: 0.25 mg PO daily; age ≥70 yrs: 0.125 mg PO daily; Renal impairment: 0.0625 to 0.125 mg PO daily. **Rapid atrial fibrillation**: Total loading dose (TLD), 10 - 15 mcg/kg IV/PO, given in 3 divided doses q 6 - 8 h; give ~50% TLD for 1 dose, then ~25% TLD for 2 doses (e.g., 70 kg with normal renal function: 0.5 mg, then 0.25 mg q 6 - 8 h for 2 doses). Impaired renal function, 6 - 10 mcg/kg IV/PO TLD, given in 3 divided doses of 0.125 - 0.375 mg IV/PO daily.	Assess electrolytes, renal function, levels periodically. Adjust dose based on response and therapeutic serum levels; recommended serum digoxin level for most patients is 0.5 to 1.0 mg/mL. The risk of adverse events increases when the serum level is more than 1.2 ng/mL. Nausea, vomiting, visual disturbances, and cardiac arrhythmias may indicate toxicity.
Digoxin Immune Fab (Digibind, DigiFab)	**Digoxin toxicity**: 1 vial binds approximately 0.5 mg digoxin. **Acute ingestion of unknown amount**: 10 vials IV, may repeat once.	Toxicity during chronic therapy: 6 vials usually adequate; one formula is: Number vials = (serum digoxin level in ng/mL) × (kg)/100.

X. Angiotensin-Converting Enzyme Inhibitors (ACE inhibitors, "-prils")

Contraindicated in pregnancy; with history of angioedema; with aliskiren in patients with DM; or with neprilysin inhibitor (e.g., sacubitril). Do not give ACE inhibitor within 36 h of switching to or from sacubitril/valsartan. In general, avoid combined use with renin-angiotensin system inhibitors (i.e., angiotensin receptor blockers, aliskiren); increases risk of renal impairment, hypotension, and hyperkalemia. Hyperkalemia possible, especially if used concomitantly with other drugs that increase K^+ (including K^+ containing salt substitutes) and in patients with DM or renal impairment. Concomitant neprilysin inhibitor (e.g., sacubitril) may increase angioedema risk. Concomitant NSAID, including celecoxib, may further deteriorate renal function and decrease antihypertensive effects.

Benazepril (Lotensin)	**HTN**: Start 10 mg PO daily, usual maintenance dose 20 to 40 mg PO daily or divided twice daily, max 80 mg/day.	
Captopril (Capoten)	**HTN**: Start 25 mg PO two to three times daily, usual maintenance dose 25 to 150 mg two to three times daily, max 450 mg/day. **Heart failure**: Start 6.25 to 12.5 mg PO three times daily, usual dose 50 to 100 mg PO three times daily, max 450 mg/day.	
Enalapril (Enalaprilat, Vasotec)	**HTN**: Start 5 mg PO daily, usual maintenance dose 10 - 40 mg PO daily or divided twice daily, max 40 mg/day. If oral therapy not possible, can use enalaprilat 1.25 mg IV q 6 h over 5 min, and increase up to 5 mg IV q 6 h if needed. Renal impairment or concomitant diuretic therapy: Start 2.5 mg PO daily. **Heart failure**: Start 2.5 mg PO twice daily, usual dose 10 - 20 mg PO twice daily, max 40 mg/day.	
Fosinopril (Monopril)	**HTN**: Start 10 mg PO daily, usual maintenance dose 20 - 40 mg PO daily or divided twice daily, max 80 mg/day. **Heart failure**: Start 5 - 10 mg PO daily, usual dose 20 - 40 mg PO daily, max 40 mg/day.	

COMMON CARDIAC DRUGS (*Continued*)		
Drug	**Dose**	**Comments**
Lisinopril (Prinivil, Zestril)	**HTN**: Start 10 mg PO daily, usual maintenance dose 20 - 40 mg PO daily, max 80 mg/day. **Heart failure**: Start 2.5 - 5 mg PO daily, usual dose 5 - 20 mg PO daily, max dose 40 mg. **Acute MI**: Give 5 mg within 24 h post MI, then 10 mg PO daily. Renal impairment (CrCl 10 - 30 mL/min): Halve the usual dose; (CrCl <10 mL/min or dialysis): Start 2.5 mg PO daily.	
Moexipril (Univasc)	**HTN**: Start 7.5 mg PO daily, usual maintenance dose 7.5 to 30 mg PO daily or divided twice daily, max 30 mg/day.	
Perindopril (Aceon, Coversyl)	**HTN**: Start 4 mg PO daily, usual maintenance dose 4 - 8 mg PO daily or divided twice daily, max 16 mg/day. **Reduction of cardiovascular events in stable CAD**: Start 4 mg PO daily for 2 weeks, max 8 mg/day. Elderly (age older than 65 yo): 4 mg PO daily, max 8 mg/day.	
Quinapril (Accupril)	**HTN**: Start 10 - 20 mg PO daily (start 10 mg/day if elderly), usual maintenance dose 20 - 80 mg PO daily or divided twice daily, max 80 mg/day. **Heart failure**: Start 5 mg PO twice daily, usual maintenance dose 10 - 20 mg twice daily.	
Ramipril (Altace)	**HTN**: 2.5 mg PO daily, usual maintenance dose 2.5 - 20 mg PO daily or divided twice daily, max 20 mg/day. **Heart failure post-MI**: Start 2.5 mg PO twice daily, usual maintenance dose 5 mg PO twice daily. **Reduce risk of MI, CVA, death from cardiovascular causes**: 2.5 mg PO daily for 1 week, then 5 mg daily for 3 weeks, increase as tolerated to max 10 mg/day.	

Trandolapril (Mavik)	**HTN**: Start 1 mg PO daily, usual maintenance dose 2 - 4 mg PO daily or divided twice daily, max 8 mg/day. **Heart failure/post-MI**: Start 1 mg PO daily, usual maintenance dose 4 mg PO daily. Renal impairment or concomitant diuretic therapy: Start 0.5 mg PO daily.	

XI. Angiotensin Receptor Antagonists (ARBs, "-sartans")

Consider as alternative if cannot tolerate ACE inhibitor (e.g., cough). Contra-indicated in pregnancy; or with aliskiren in patients with DM. In general, avoid combined use with renin-angiotensin system inhibitors (i.e., ACE inhibitors, aliskiren, sacubitril/valsartan); increases risk of renal impairment, hypotension, and hyperkalemia. Hyperkalemia possible, especially if used concomitantly with other drugs that increase K^+ (including K^+ containing salt substitutes) and in patients with heart failure, DM, or renal impairment. Concomitant NSAID, including celecoxib, may further deteriorate renal function and decrease anti-hypertensive effects.

Azilsartan (Edarbi)	**HTN**: 80 mg PO daily.	
Candesartan (Atacand)	**HTN**: Start 16 mg PO daily, max 32 mg/day. **Heart failure (NYHA II–IV and LVEF 40% or less)**: Start 4 mg PO daily, max 32 mg/day. Renal impairment (mild-moderate): Start 8 mg PO day; do not use if GFR < 30 mL/min/1.73 m2.	
Eprosartan (Teveten)	**HTN**: Start 600 mg PO daily, max 900 mg/day given daily or divided twice daily. Renal impairment (CrCl <30 mL/min): Max 600 mg/day.	
Irbesartan (Avapro)	**HTN**: Start 150 mg PO daily, max 300 mg/day.	
Losartan (Cozaar)	**HTN**: Start 50 mg PO daily; max 100 mg/day given daily or divided twice daily. **Volume-depleted patients or history of hepatic impairment**: Start 25 mg PO daily.	

COMMON CARDIAC DRUGS (*Continued*)		
Drug	**Dose**	**Comments**
Olmesartan (Benicar, Olmetec)	**HTN**: Start 20 mg PO daily; max 40 mg/day.	
Telmisartan (Micardis)	**HTN**: Start 40 mg PO daily; max 80 mg/day. **Cardiovascular risk reduction**: Start 80 mg PO daily, max 80 mg/day.	
Valsartan (Diovan)	**HTN**: Start 80 - 160 mg PO daily, max 320 mg/day. **Heart failure**: Start 40 mg PO twice daily, target dose 160 mg twice daily. **Reduce mortality/morbidity post-MI with LV systolic dysfunction/ failure**: Start 20 mg PO twice daily, target dose 160 mg twice daily.	

XII. Angiotensin Receptor Neprilysin Inhibitor ("ARNI")

Usually given with other heart failure therapies, in place of ACE inhibitor or other ARB. If switching from ACE inhibitor, allow 36 h washout period between administration of the drugs. Do not use with severe hepatic impairment or inherited angioedema. Contraindicated with pregnancy, concomitant ACE inhibitor, concomitant aliskiren in patients with DM, or previous angioedema with ACE inhibitor or angiotensin receptor blocker. Combined use with renin-angiotensin system inhibitors (i.e., ACE inhibitors, aliskiren, other angiotensin receptor blocker) increases risk of renal impairment, hypotension, and hyperkalemia. Hyperkalemia possible, especially if used concomitantly with other drugs that increase K^+ (including K^+-containing salt substitutes) and in patients with heart failure, DM, or renal impairment. Concomitant NSAID, including celecoxib, may further deteriorate renal function and decrease antihypertensive effects.

Entresto (Sacubitril + Valsartan)	**Heart failure (NYHA Class II–IV) with reduced EF**: Start 49/51 mg PO twice daily, double dose after 2 - 4 weeks as tolerated, target maintenance dose 97/103 mg PO twice daily. Patients not currently taking ACE inhibitor or ARB or previously taking low dose of these agents, severe renal impairment (eGFR < 30 mL/min/1.73 m^2), moderate hepatic impairment: Start 24/26 mg PO twice daily, double dose after 2 - 4 weeks as tolerated; target dose 97/103 mg PO twice daily.	

XIII. Direct Renin Inhibitor

Contraindicated in pregnancy; or with ACEi or ARBs in patients with DM. Avoid use with ACEi or ARBs, particularly in patients with CrCl <60 mL/min; increases risk of renal impairment, hypotension, and hyperkalemia. Concomitant NSAID, including celecoxib, may further deteriorate renal function and decrease antihypertensive effects. Hyperkalemia possible, especially if used concomitantly with other drugs that increase K^+ (including K^+-containing salt substitutes) and in patients with heart failure, DM, or renal impairment. Monitor potassium and renal function periodically.

Aliskiren (Tekturna)	HTN: 150 mg PO daily, max 300 mg/day.	

XIV. Loop Diuretics

Thiazides are preferred diuretics for HTN. With decreased renal function (CrCl <30 mL/min), loop diuretics may be more effective than thiazides for HTN. Rare hypersensitivity in patients allergic to sulfa-containing drugs, except ethacrynic acid. For diuretics given twice daily, give second dose in midafternoon to avoid nocturia.

Bumetanide (Bumex, Burinex)	Edema: 0.5 - 1 mg IV/IM; 0.5 to 2 mg PO daily.	1 mg bumetanide = 40 mg furosemide = 20 mg torsemide
Ethacrynic acid (Edecrin)	Edema: 0.5 - 1 mg/kg IV, max 100 mg/dose; 25 to 100 mg PO daily to twice daily.	Can be safely used in patients with true sulfa allergy.
Furosemide (Lasix)	HTN: Start 10 - 40 mg PO twice daily, max 600 mg daily. Edema: Start 20 - 80 mg IV/IM/ PO, increase dose by 20 to 40 mg in 6 - 8 h until desired response is achieved, max 600 mg/ day.	
Torsemide (Demadex)	HTN: Start 5 mg PO daily, increase prn q 4 - 6 weeks, max 10 mg daily. Edema: 10 - 20 mg IV/PO daily, max 200 mg IV/PO daily.	

COMMON CARDIAC DRUGS (*Continued*)

Drug	Dose	Comments
XV. Thiazide Diuretics Possible hypersensitivity in sulfa allergy. Should be used for most patients with HTN, alone or combined with other antihypertensive agents. With decreased renal function (CrCl <30 mL/min), loop diuretics may be more effective than thiazides for HTN. Thiazides are not recommended for gestational HTN. Coadministration with NSAIDs, including selective COX-2 inhibitors, may reduce the antihypertensive, diuretic, and natriuretic effects of thiazides. May use thiazide in combination with oral potassium supplementation, ACE inhibitor, ARB, or potassium-sparing diuretic to maintain K level.		
Chlorothiazide (Diuril)	**HTN:** Start 125-250 mg PO daily or divided twice daily, max 1000 mg/day divided twice daily.	
Chlorthalidone (Hygroton)	**HTN:** 12.5 - 25 mg PO daily, max 50 mg/day. **Edema:** 50 - 100 mg PO daily, max 200 mg/day.	Chlorthalidone is preferred on the basis of prolonged half-life and proven trial reduction of cardiovascular disease.
Hydrochlorothiazide (HCTZ, Microzide)	**HTN:** 12.5 - 25 mg PO daily, max 50 mg/day. **Edema:** 25 - 100 mg PO daily, max 200 mg/day.	
Indapamide (Lozol)	**HTN:** 1.25 - 5 mg PO daily, max 5 mg/day. **Edema:** 2.5 - 5 mg PO q am.	
Metolazone (Zaroxolyn)	**Edema:** 5 - 10 mg PO daily, max 10 mg/day in heart failure, 20 mg/day in renal disease. If used with loop diuretic, start with 2.5 mg PO daily.	

XVI. Aldosterone Antagonists

Hyperkalemia possible, especially if used concomitantly with other drugs that increase K (including K-containing salt substitutes) and in patients with heart failure, DM, or renal impairment.

Eplerenone (Inspra)	**HTN**: Start 50 mg PO daily; max 50 mg twice daily. **Heart failure (with LVEF 40% or less) post MI**: Start 25 mg PO daily; titrate to target dose 50 mg daily within 4 weeks, if tolerated.	Contraindicated in all patients with $K^+ > 5.5$ mEq/L; CrCl ≤ 30 mL/min. Contraindicated in patients treated for HTN with Type 2 DM with microalbuminuria; serum Cr > 2 mg/dL in males or > 1.8 mg/dL in females; CrCl < 50 mL/min; or concomitant therapy with K^+ supplements, K^+-sparing diuretics. Hyperkalemia is more common with renal impairment, diabetes, proteinuria, or with ACEi, ARB, or NSAID.
Spironolactone (Aldactone)	**HTN**: 50 - 100 mg PO daily or divided twice daily (usual dose 25 - 50 mg daily according to ASH-ISH guidelines). **Edema**: 25 - 200 mg/day. **Heart failure, NYHA III or IV**: 25 to 50 mg PO daily.	Use with caution when SCr > 2.5 mg/dL or $K^+ > 5$ mEq/L. This is a preferred agent in primary aldosteronism and resistant hypertension. Greater risk of gynecomastia and impotence as compared with Epleronone.
XVII. Inotropes and Vasopressors		
Dobutamine (Dobutrex)	**Inotropic support**: Start 0.5 - 1 mcg/kg/min; titrate based on response; usual dose 2 - 20 mcg/kg/min.	Stimulates $\beta1$, $\beta2$, and α receptors.
Dopamine (Intropin)	**Pressor**: Start at 5 mcg/kg/min, increase prn by 5 - 10 mcg/kg/min increments at 10-min intervals, max 50 mcg/kg/min.	Doses in mcg/kg/min: 2 - 5 (renal dose) dopaminergic receptors; 5 - 10 (cardiac dose) dopaminergic and β-1 receptors; > 10 dopaminergic, β-1, and α-1 receptors.

COMMON CARDIAC DRUGS (*Continued*)

Drug	Dose	Comments
Epinephrine (EpiPen, EpiPen Jr, Adrenalin)	**Cardiac arrest**: 1 mg IV q 3 - 5 min.	
Midodrine (Amatine)	**Orthostatic hypotension**: 10 mg PO three times daily.	The last daily dose should be no later than 6 pm to avoid supine HTN during sleep. Avoid concomitant medications that increase BP (eg., dihydroergotamine, ephedrine, phenylephrine, pseudoephedrine, thyroid hormones), or MAO inhibitors.
Milrinone (Primacor)	**Systolic heart failure (NYHA class III, IV)**: Load 50 mcg/kg IV over 10 min, then begin IV infusion of 0.375 - 0.75 mcg/kg/min.	Phosphodiesterase-3 inhibitor.
Norepinephrine (Levophed)	**Acute hypotension**: Start 8 to 12 mcg/min, adjust to maintain BP, average maintenance rate 2 - 4 mcg/min.	Ideally through central line.
Phenylephrine (NeoSynephrine)	**Severe hypotension**: Start 100 to 180 mcg/min (75 to 135 mL/h), usual dose once BP is stabilized 40 to 60 mcg/min.	

XVIII. Antiarrhythmic Agents

Drug	Dose	Comments
Adenosine (Adenocard)	**PSVT conversion (not Atrial fibrillation)**: 6 mg rapid IV push and flush. If no response after 1 - 2 min, then 12 mg. A 3rd dose of 12 mg may be given prn.	Half-life is less than 10 sec. Give doses by rapid IV push followed by NS flush. Need higher dose if on theophylline or caffeine, lower dose if on dipyridamole.

Amiodarone (Pacerone, Cordarone)	**Life-threatening ventricular arrhythmia without cardiac arrest**: Load 150 mg IV over 10 min, then 1 mg/min for 6 h, then 0.5 mg/min for 18 h. Mix in D5W. Oral loading dose 800 - 1600 mg PO daily for 1 - 3 weeks, reduce to 400 - 800 mg PO daily for 1 month when arrhythmia is controlled, reduce to lowest effective dose thereafter, usually 200 - 400 mg PO daily.	Hypersensitivity pneumonitis, pulmonary alveolitis, sinus bradycardia, conduction abnormalities, ↑QT interval, torsades de pointes (<1%), thyroid abnormalities, corneal deposits, optic neuritis, tremor, ataxia, peripheral neuropathy, blue-gray skin discoloration, photosensitivity, nausea, ↓appetite, ↑LFT. May increase digoxin levels; discontinue digoxin or decrease dose by 50%. May increase INR with warfarin; decrease warfarin dose by 33 to 50%. Do not use with grapefruit juice. Do not use with simvastatin dose greater than 20 mg/day, lovastatin dose greater than 40 mg/ day; may increase atorvastatin level; increases risk of myopathy and rhabdomyolysis.
Atropine (AtroPen)	**Bradyarrhythmia/CPR**: 0.5 to 1 mg IV q 3 to 5 min to max 0.04 mg/kg (3 mg).	
Disopyramide (Norpace, Norpace CR)	**Ventricular arrhythmia**: 400 -800 mg PO daily in divided doses (immediate-release is divided q 6 h: extended-release is divided q 12 h).	Proarrhythmia, increased QT, torsades de pointes. Anticholinergic side effects

COMMON CARDIAC DRUGS (*Continued*)		
Drug	**Dose**	**Comments**
Dofetilide (Tikosyn)	**Atrial fibrillation/flutter conversion**: dosing based on CrCl and QTc interval. CrCl > 60 mL/min: 500 mcg twice daily; CrCl 40 - 60 mL/min: 250 mcg twice daily; CrCl 20 - 40 mL/min: 125 mcg twice daily; Contraindicated in patients with CrCI < 20 mL/min or if baseline QTc exceeds 440 ms (or if baseline QTc > 500 msec in patients with ventricular conduction abnormalities)	Measure QTc 2-3 hr after the first dose. If no significant QTc prolongation is observed, the drug should be continued at the initial dose. If QTc increases by > 15% or if QTc exceeds 500 msec, (550 msec in patients with ventricular conduction abnormalities) the drug should be decreased by half.
Dronedarone (Multaq)	**Maintain sinus rhythm for Atrial fibrillation**: 400 mg PO twice daily with morning and evening meals.	May initiate or worsen heart failure symptoms. Decrease side effects/efficacy compared to amiodarone. May cause hepatic injury. Monitor renal function. May increase INR when used with warfarin. May increase dabigatran level. May increase digoxin level; discontinue digoxin or decrease dose by 50%. Use caution with β-blockers (BB) and calcium channel blockers (CCB); initiate lower doses of BB or CCB and monitor ECG. Do not use with > 10 mg of simvastatin. Do not use with permanent A fib, NYHA Class IV heart failure or NYHA Class II - III heart failure with recent decompensation, 2nd or 3rd degree AV block or SSS without pacemaker, bradycardia < 50 bpm, QTc >500 msec, liver or lung toxicity related to amiodarone, severe hepatic impairment, pregnancy, grapefruit juice, drugs that increase QT interval, or Class I or III antiarrhythmic agents.

Flecainide (Tambocor)	**Prevention of paroxysmal atrial fib/flutter or PSVT, with symptoms and no structural heart disease**: Start 50 mg PO q 12 h, may increase by 50 mg twice daily q 4 days, max 300 mg/day. **Life-threatening ventricular arrhythmias without structural heart disease**: Start 100 mg PO q 12 h, may increase by 50 mg twice daily q 4 days, max 400 mg/day. With CrCl < 35 mL/min: Start 50 mg PO twice daily.	Use with AV nodal slowing agent (beta-blocker, verapamil, diltiazem) to minimize risk of 1:1 atrial flutter. Do not give if structural/ischemic heart disease.
Ibutilide (Corvert)	**Recent onset A-fib/flutter**: 0.01 mg/kg up to 1 mg IV over 10 min, may repeat once if no response after 10 min.	Keep on cardiac monitor at least 4 h.
Isoproterenol (Isuprel)	**Refractory bradycardia or 3rd degree AV block**: bolus method: 0.02 to 0.06 mg IV; infusion method: 5 mcg/min.	
Ivabradine (Corlanor)	Stable, symptomatic heart failure with reduced EF ≤35%, sinus rhythm with HR ≥70 bpm, and maximally tolerated β-blocker or intolerant to β-blocker: Start 5 mg PO twice daily; max 15 mg/day.	With conduction defect or if bradycardia could lead to hemodynamic compromise, start 2.5 mg PO two times daily. Contraindicated with acute decompensated heart failure; BP < 90/50 mmHg; resting heart rate less than 60 bpm prior to treatment; sick sinus syndrome, sinoatrial block, or 3rd degree AV block without functioning pacemaker; severe hepatic impairment; or pacemaker dependent.

COMMON CARDIAC DRUGS (*Continued*)		
Drug	**Dose**	**Comments**
Lidocaine (Xylocaine)	**Ventricular arrhythmia**: Load 1 mg/kg IV, then 0.5 mg/kg q 8 - 10 min prn to max 3 mg/kg.	
Mexiletine (Mexitil)	**Ventricular arrhythmia**: Start 200 mg PO q 8 h with food or antacid, max dose 1200 mg/day. Renal impairment (CrCl ≤10 mL/min): Use 50 to 75% of dose.	
Procainamide (Procan, Pronestyl)	**Ventricular arrhythmia**: Loading dose: 100 mg IV q10 min or 20 mg/min (150 mL/h) until QRS widens more than 50%, dysrhythmia suppressed, hypotension, or total of 17 mg/kg or 1000 mg delivered. **Rapid atrial fibrillation with preexcitation (WPW)**: Start 15 - 17 mg/kg IV x 1 or 100 mg IV q 5 - 10 min, max 1.5 gram; maintenance 9 gram/day.	Associated with lupus-like syndrome. Proarrhythmia, increased QT, torsades de pointes.
Propafenone (Rythmol, Rythmol SR)	**Prevention of paroxysmal A-fib/flutter or PSVT, with symptoms and no structural heart disease; or life-threatening ventricular arrhythmias**: Start (immediate-release) 150 mg PO q 8 h, may increase after 3 - 4 days to 225 mg PO q 8 h, max 900 mg/day. **Prolong time to recurrence of symptomatic A-fib without structural heart disease**: 225 mg SR PO q 12 h, may increase after 5 days to 325 mg SR PO q 12 h, max 425 mg SR PO q 12 h.	Consider using with AV nodal blocking agent (beta-blocker, verapamil, diltiazem) to minimize risk of 1:1 atrial flutter. Do not use with amiodarone or quinidine. May increase digoxin, warfarin, beta-blocker levels.

Quinidine (Quinaglute, Quinidex, Cardioquin)	**Conversion/prevention of atrial fibrillation/flutter, ventricular tachycardia**: Gluconate, extended-release: 324 - 648 mg PO q 8 to 12 h; sulfate, immediate-release: 200 - 400 mg PO q 6 - 8 h; sulfate, extended-release: 300 - 600 mg PO q 8 - 12 h.	Proarrhythmia, increased QT, torsades de pointes. Cinchonism (tinnitus, hearing loss)
Sotalol (Betapace, Betapace AF)	**Ventricular arrhythmia** (Betapace): Start 80 mg PO twice daily, max 640 mg/day. **Atrial fibrillation/flutter** (Betapace AF): Start 80 mg PO twice daily, max 640 mg/day.	Proarrhythmia, increased QT, torsades de pointes. Should not be initiated as outpatient if structural heart disease present.

XIX. HMG-CoA Reductase Inhibitors ("Statins")

Measure creatinine kinase before starting statin if patient at risk for adverse muscle events. Risk of myopathy increases with advanced age (≥65 yrs), female gender, uncontrolled hypothyroidism, renal dysfunction, higher statin doses, and concomitant use of certain medications (e.g., fibrates, niacin, or ranolazine). Check liver function (e.g., ALT, AST) before starting statin and as clinically indicated thereafter. Discontinue statin with persistent ALT elevations more than 3 times the upper limit of normal or objective evidence of liver injury. Measure HbA1c before starting statin if diabetes status unknown. Statins may increase the risk of hyperglycemia and type 2 diabetes; benefit outweighs risk. No clear evidence that statins adversely affect cognition. If patient complains of confusion or memory impairment while on statin therapy, consider other possible etiologies, including certain drugs (e.g., sleeping pills, analgesics) and medical conditions (e.g., depression, anxiety, obstructive sleep apnea) that affect memory.

Atorvastatin (Lipitor)	**Hyperlipidemia/prevention of cardiovascular events**: Start 10 - 40 mg PO daily, max 80 mg/day.	Do not exceed 20 mg/day when given with clarithromycin, itraconazole, or other HIV protease inhibitors.
Fluvastatin (Lescol, Lescol XL)	**Hyperlipidemia**: Start 20 - 80 mg PO q HS, max 80 mg daily (XL) or divided twice daily.	

COMMON CARDIAC DRUGS (*Continued*)		
Drug	**Dose**	**Comments**
Lovastatin (Mevacor)	**Hyperlipidemia/prevention of cardiovascular events**: Start 20 mg PO q pm, max 80 mg/day daily or divided twice daily.	Do not use with clarithromycin, erythromycin, gemfibrozil, grapefruit juice, HIV protease inhibitors, itraconazole, or ketoconazole; increases risk of myopathy. Do not exceed 20 mg/day when used with diltiazem, dronedarone, verapamil, or CrCl <30 mL/min. Do not exceed 40 mg/day when used with amiodarone.
Pitavastatin (Livalo)	**Hyperlipidemia**: Start 2 mg PO at bedtime, max 4 mg daily. CrCl 15 - 59 mL/min or on dialysis: Start 1 mg PO daily, max 2 mg daily.	Do not exceed 2 mg/day when given with rifampin.
Pravastatin (Pravachol)	**Hyperlipidemia/prevention of cardiovascular events**: Start 40 mg PO daily, max 80 mg/day.	Lowest risk of myopathy and safest in liver disease compared to other statins.
Rosuvastatin (Crestor)	**Hyperlipidemia/slow progression of atherosclerosis/ primary prevention of CVD**: Start 10 - 20 mg PO daily, max 40 mg/day. Renal impairment (CrCl <30 mL/min and not on hemodialysis): Start 5 mg PO daily, max 10 mg/day. Asians: Start 5 mg PO daily.	When given with HIV protease inhibitors (e.g. atazanavir ritonavir, lopinavir), do not exceed 10 mg/day. Avoid using with gemfibrozil; if used concomitantly, do not exceed 10 mg/day.

Simvastatin (Zocor)	**Hyperlipidemia**: Start 10 - 20 mg PO q HS, max 40 mg/day. **Reduce cardiovascular mortality/events in high risk for coronary heart disease event**: Start 40 mg PO q pm, max 40 mg/day. Severe renal impairment: Start 5 mg/day, closely monitor.	Do not initiate therapy with or titrate to 80 mg/day; only use 80 mg/day in patients who have taken this dose for more than 12 months without evidence of muscle toxicity. Do not use with clarithromycin, erythromycin, gemfibrozil, grapefruit juice, HIV protease inhibitors, itraconazole, ketoconazole; increases risk of myopathy. Do not exceed 10 mg/day when used with diltiazem, dronedarone, or verapamil. Do not exceed 20 mg/day when used with amiodarone, amlodipine or ranolazine.

XX. Bile Acid Sequestrants

Cholestyramine (Questran, Questran Light)	**Elevated LDL-C**: Powder: Start 4 g PO daily to twice daily before meals, increase up to max 24 g/day.	Causes GI distress, constipation, bloating.
Colesevelam (Welchol, Lodalis)	**LDL-C reduction or glycemic control of type 2 diabetes**: 3.75 g once daily or 1.875 g PO twice daily, max 3.75 g/day.	Causes GI distress, constipation, bloating.
Colestipol (Colestid, Colestid Flavored)	**Elevated LDL-C**: Tabs: Start 2 g PO daily to twice daily, max 16 g/day. Granules: Start 5 g PO daily to twice daily, max 30 g/day.	Causes GI distress, constipation, bloating.

COMMON CARDIAC DRUGS (*Continued*)

Drug	Dose	Comments
XXI. Fibrates		

Contraindicated with liver disease, gall bladder disease, and/or severe renal impairment. Evaluate renal function at baseline, within 3 months after initiation, q 6 months thereafter. Monitor LFTs (baseline, periodically). Use in combination with statin therapy is not proven to reduce risk of CV events beyond statin monotherapy. Increased risk of myopathy and rhabdomyolysis when used with a statin. May increase cholesterol excretion into bile, leading to cholelithiasis. May increase the effect of warfarin.

Drug	Dose	Comments
Fenofibrate (TriCor, Antara, Fenoglide, Lipofen, Triglide, Lipidil Micro, Lipidil Supra, Lipidil EZ)	**Hypertriglyceridemia**: <u>TriCor tabs</u>: 48 - 145 mg PO daily, max 145 mg daily. **Hypercholesterolemia/mixed dyslipidemia**: <u>TriCor tabs</u>: 145 mg PO daily. Reduce dose for mild to moderate renal insufficiency.	May consider concomitant therapy with a low- or moderate-intensity statin if the benefits from triglyceride lowering (when ≥500 mg/dL) outweigh the risk of adverse effects. May increase serum creatinine level without changing eGFR.
Fenofibric acid (Trilipix)	**Hypertriglyceridemia**: <u>Trilipix</u>: 45 - 135 mg PO daily, max 135 mg daily. **Hypercholesterolemia/mixed dyslipidemia**: <u>Trilipix</u>: 135mg PO daily. Renal impairment: TriLipix: 45 mg PO daily.	May increase serum creatinine level without changing eGFR.
Gemfibrozil (Lopid)	**Hypertriglyceridemia/primary prevention of CAD**: 600 mg PO twice daily 30 min before meals.	Do not use with statin; increases risk of myopathy and rhabdomyolysis.
XXII. Nicotinic Acid		
Niacin (vitamin B3, nicotinic acid, Slo-Niacin, Niaspan)	**Hyperlipidemia**: Start 50 - 100 mg PO two to three times daily with meals, increase slowly, usual maintenance range 1.5 - 3 g/day, max 6 g/day. Extended-release (<u>Niaspan</u>): Start 500 mg at bedtime, increase monthly up to max 2000 mg. Extended-release formulations may have greater hepatotoxicity.	Start with low doses and increase slowly to minimize flushing; 325 mg aspirin (non-EC) 30 - 60 min prior to niacin ingestion will minimize flush.

XXIII. Omega Fatty Acids

FDA-approved medication with purified omega-3 fatty acids from fish oils. Lovaza may paradoxically increase LDL-C in patients with very high triglyceride values, but Vascepa apparently does not. May prolong bleeding time, may potentiate warfarin. Monitor AST/ALT if hepatic impairment. Use caution in patients with known hypersensitivity to fish and/or shellfish.

Icosapent ethyl (Vascepa)	**Hypertriglyceridemia** (500 mg/dL or above): 2 g PO twice daily.	Contains EPA. May reduce cardiovascular risk (FDA-approved for this indication)
Omega-3-acid ethyl esters (Lovaza)	**Hypertriglyceridemia** (≥500 mg/dL): 4 caps PO daily or divided twice daily.	Contains EPA + DHA.

XXIV. Proprotein convertase subtilisin/kexin type 9 (PCSK-9) Inhibitors

Alirocumab (Praluent)	**Reduce LDL-C as adjunct to diet and maximally tolerated statin with heterozygous familial hypercholesterolemia or clinical atherosclerotic CVD**: Start 75 mg SC q 2 weeks, max 150 mg q 2 weeks; or 300 mg SC q 4 weeks (monthly). To give 300 mg dose, inject 2 doses of 150 mg consecutively at two different injection sites.	Human monoclonal antibody. Give in abdomen, upper arm, or thigh. May consider in very high risk ASCVD patients if LDL-cholesterol ≥ 70 mg/dL on maximally tolerated statin therapy.
Evolocumab (Repatha)	**Secondary prevention for patients with established cardiovascular disease**: 140 mg SC q 2 weeks or 420 mg SQ once monthly. **Reduce LDL-C as adjunct to diet alone or in combination with other lipid-lowering therapies for primary hyperlipidemia**: 140 mg SC every 2 weeks or 420 mg SQ once monthly. **Reduce LDL-C as adjunct to diet and other lipid lowering therapies for patients with homozygous familial hypercholesterolemia**: 420 mg SQ once monthly.	Human monoclonal antibody. Give in abdomen, upper arm, or thigh. May consider in very high risk ASCVD patients if LDL-cholesterol ≥ 70 mg/dL on maximally tolerated statin therapy.

COMMON CARDIAC DRUGS (*Continued*)

Drug	Dose	Comments
XXV. Cholesterol Absorption Inhibitor		
Ezetimibe (Zetia)	**Hyperlipidemia**: 10 mg PO daily.	May consider in very high risk ASCVD patients if LDL-cholesterol ≥ 70 mg/dL on maximally tolerated statin therapy.

XXVI. α-1 Antagonists
These are associated with orthostatic hypotension, especially in older adults. They may be considered as second-line agent for HTN in patients with concomitant BPH. Avoid if patient takes PDE-5 inhibitor (e.g., sildenafil, tadalafil, vardenafil) due to increased risk of hypotension.

Drug	Dose	Comments
Doxazosin (Cardura, Cardura XL)	**HTN, immediate-release:** Start 1 mg PO at bedtime, max 16 mg/day.	Take 1st dose at bedtime to minimize orthostatic hypotension.
Prazosin (Minipress)	**HTN**: Start 1 mg PO two to three times daily, max 40 mg/day.	Take 1st dose at bedtime to minimize orthostatic hypotension.
Terazosin (Hytrin)	**HTN**: Start 1 mg PO at bedtime, usual effective dose 1 - 5 mg PO daily or divided twice daily, max 20 mg/day.	Take 1st dose at bedtime to minimize orthostatic hypotension.

XXVII. Central α-2 Receptor Agonists and Other Centrally Acting Drugs
Generally last-line agent for hypertension (HTN) because of significant CNS adverse effects, especially in older adults. Avoid abrupt discontinuation of clonidine, which may induce hypertensive crisis.

Drug	Dose	Comments
Clonidine (Catapres, Catapres TTS)	**HTN, immediate-release:** Start 0.1 mg PO twice daily, usual maintenance dose 0.2 - 0.6 mg/day in 2 - 3 divided doses, max 2.4 mg daily. Rebound HTN with abrupt discontinuation, taper dose slowly. **HTN,** transdermal (Catapres-TTS): Start 0.1 mg/24 h patch once a week, titrate to desired effect, max effective dose 0.6 mg/24 h (two 0.3 mg/24h patches).	May cause dizziness, drowsiness, or lightheadedness. Monitor for bradycardia when taking concomitant digitalis, non-dihydropyridine calcium channel blockers, or beta-blockers. Renal impairment: Consider using a lower initial dose; monitor for bradycardia, hypotension, and sedation.

Fenoldopam (Corlopam)	**Severe HTN**: Start at 0.1 mcg/kg/min, titrate q 15 min, usual effective dose 0.1 - 1.6 mcg/kg/min.	
Guanfacine (Tenex)	**HTN**: Start 1 mg PO at bedtime, may increase by 1 mg at bedtime every 3 - 4 weeks, max 3 mg/day. Renal impairment (<30 mL/min): Use lower dose; monitor closely for side effects.	
Methyldopa (Aldomet)	**HTN**: Start 250 mg PO 2 - 3 times daily, max 3000 mg/day. Renal impairment (CrCl 10 - 50 mL/min): give q 8 - 12 h; (<10 mL/min): give q 12 - 24 h.	May be used to manage HTN during pregnancy.

XXVIII. Direct Vasodilators

These are associated with sodium and water retention and reflex tachycardia; use with a diuretic and beta blocker.

Hydralazine (Apresoline)	**Hypertensive emergency**: 10 - 20 mg IV or 10 - 50 mg IM, repeat prn. **HTN**: Start 10 mg PO two to four times daily, max 300 mg/day.	Associated with lupus-like syndrome at higher doses. Vascular smooth muscle-mediated peripheral vasodilation
Hydralazine + Isosorbide dinitrate (Bidil)	**Heart failure** (adjunct therapy in black patients): Start 1 tab (37.5/20 mg) PO three times daily, increase as tolerated to max 2 tabs three times daily. May decrease to ½ tab three times daily with intolerable side effects.	Consider if cannot tolerate ACE inhibitor/ARB in black patients with heart failure

COMMON CARDIAC DRUGS (*Continued*)

Drug	Dose	Comments
Minoxidil (Loniten)	**Refractory HTN**: Start 2.5 - 5 mg PO daily, increase at no less than 3-day intervals, usual dose 10 - 40 mg daily, max 100 mg/day.	Relatively contraindicated in patients with coronary disease (i.e., recent/acute MI, angina, renal disease, pulmonary hypertension, or chronic heart failure not secondary to HTN (drug may increase pulmonary artery pressure). Associated with hirsutism and requires a loop diuretic. Can induce pericardial effusion.
Nesiritide (Natrecor)	**CHF, acutely decompensated**: start 2 mcg/kg IV x1, then 0.01 mcg/kg/min IV; max 0.03 mcg/kg/min. May increase by 0.005 mcg/kg/min IV q3h; decrease dose or D/C if symptomatic hypotension, may restart without bolus at 30% lower dose	For patients with dyspnea at rest or minimal exertion.
Nitroprusside (Nipride, Nitropress)	**Hypertensive emergency**: start 0.3 mcg/kg/min. Max 10 mcg/kg/min.	Protect from light. Cyanide toxicity with high doses (10 mcg/kg/min), hepatic/renal impairment, and prolonged infusions (longer than 3 - 7 days); check thiocyanate levels.
XXIX. Other Claudication Drugs		
Pentoxifylline (Trental)	**Intermittent claudication**: 400 mg PO three times daily with meals.	Contraindicated with recent cerebral/retinal bleed. Lowers blood viscosity and improves erythrocyte flexibility

XXXa. Pulmonary Artery Hypertension (PAH) Drugs: Endothelin Receptor Antagonists ("-sentans")

Patients with LV dysfunction may develop significant fluid retention and worsening heart failure after initiating endothelin receptor antagonist therapy; monitor for signs and symptoms of fluid retention.

Ambrisentan (Letairis)	**PAH**: Start 5 mg PO daily; max 10 mg/day; titrate q 4 weeks as needed and tolerated.	May give with Tadalafil to improve exercise ability and decrease disease progression and hospitalizations. Contraindicated with idiopathic pulmonary fibrosis or pregnancy.
Bosentan (Tracleer)	**PAH**: Start 62.5 mg PO twice daily x 4 weeks, increase to 125 mg twice daily maintenance	Hepatotoxicity; monitor LFTs. Contraindicated in pregnancy.
Macitentan (Opsumit)	**PAH**: 10 mg PO daily.	Contraindicated with pregnancy. Monitor liver function test before initiating therapy and as clinically indicated thereafter.

XXXb. Pulmonary Artery Hypertension Drugs: Phosphodiesterase Type-5 Inhibitors ("-afils")

Seek medical attention for vision loss, hearing loss, or in men if erections last > 4 h.

Sildenafil (Revatio)	**PAH**: 5 mg or 20 mg PO three times daily, with doses 4 to 6 h apart; or 2.5 mg or 10 mg IV three times daily.	Contraindicated with nitrates or guanylate cyclase stimulators (e.g., Riociguat). Coadministration is not recommended with Ritonavir, potent CYP3A4 inhibitors, or other phosphodiesterase-5 inhibitors.
Tadalafil (Adcirca)	PAH: 40 mg PO daily.	Contraindicated with nitrates or guanylate cyclase stimulators (e.g., Riociguat). Coadministration is not recommended with potent CYP3A inhibitors (Itraconazole, Ketoconazole), potent CYP3A inducers (rifampin), other phosphodiesterase-5 inhibitors. Caution with ritonavir.

COMMON CARDIAC DRUGS (*Continued*)

Drug	Dose	Comments
XXXc. Pulmonary Artery Hypertension Drugs: Prostanoids		
Epoprostenol (Flolan, Veletri)	**PAH**: Start 2 ng/kg/min IV infusion via central venous catheter.	Avoid abrupt dose decreases or cessation.
Iloprost (Ventavis)	**PAH**: Start 2.5 mcg/dose by inhalation (as delivered at mouthpiece); if well tolerated, increase to 5 mcg/dose by inhalation (as delivered at mouthpiece). Use 6 - 9 times daily (minimum of 2 h between doses) while awake.	Monitor vital signs when initiating therapy. Do not initiate therapy if SBP less than 85 mmHg. May induce bronchospasm.
Selexipag (Uptravi)	**PAH**: Start 200 mcg PO twice daily, increase by 200 mcg PO twice daily each week to highest tolerated dose, max 1600 mcg PO twice daily. With moderate hepatic impairment (Childs-Pugh class B): Start 200 mcg PO daily, increase by 200 mcg PO daily each week to highest tolerated dose, max 1600 mcg PO daily.	Avoid with severe hepatic impairment. Contraindicated with strong CYP2C8 inhibitors (e.g. gemfibrozil).
Treprostinil (Remodulin – IV, Tyvaso – Inhaled, Orenitram – oral)	**PAH**: (Remodulin – IV) Continuous SC (preferred) or central IV infusion. Start 1.25 ng/kg/min based on ideal body wt. Dose based on clinical response and tolerance. (Tyvaso – Inhaled) Start 3 breaths (18 mcg) per treatment session four times daily while awake; treatments should be at least 4 h apart; max 9 breaths (54 mcg) per treatment four times daily. Administer undiluted with the Tyvaso Inhalation System. (Orenitram – oral) Start 0.25 mg PO two times daily; increase by 0.25 - 0.5 mg two times daily or 0.125 mg three times daily q 3 - 4 days as tolerated. To transition from IV or SC treprostinil, simultaneously decrease IV/SC infusion rate up to 30 ng/kg/min per day and increase the oral treprostinil dose up to 6 mg per day (2 mg three times daily).	Avoid abruptly lowering the dose or cessation. Use cautiously in the elderly and those with liver or renal dysfunction. Administer by continuous infusion using infusion pump. Inhibits platelet aggregation; may increase bleeding risk. May potentiate bleeding risk for patients on anticoagulants. May potentiate hypotensive effects of other medications.

XXXc. Pulmonary Artery Hypertension Drugs: Soluble Guanylate Cyclase Stimulator

Riociguat (Adempas)	**PAH**: Start 1 mg PO three times daily; max 2.5 mg three times daily.	Contraindicated with pregnancy, nitrates, nitric oxide donors, PDE-5 inhibitors (e.g., sildenafil, tadalafil, vardenafil), nonspecific PDE inhibitors (e.g., dipyridamole, theophylline).

Note: Adapted from prescribing information; Antman, EM (ed) Cardiovascular Therapeutics: A Companion to Braunwald's Heart Disease 3rd ed., 2006; Hamilton RJ (ed), Tarascon Pocket Pharmacopoeia, 2019; Sabatine, MS (ed) Pocket Medicine 6th ed., 2017; Epocrates®, 2019; 2017 ACC/AHA Guideline for High Blood Pressure; 2013 ACCF/AHA Guideline for Heart Failure; 2017 ACC/AHA Focused Update of the Guideline for Heart Failure; 2011 ACCF/AHA Guideline for PCI; 2014 ACC/AHA Focused Update of the Guideline for SIHD; 2012 ACCF/AHA Guideline for SIHD; ACC/AHA 2017 Appropriate Use Criteria for Coronary Revascularization in SIHD; 2014 AHA/ACC Guideline for NSTE-ACS; 2015 ACC/AHA Focused Update on Primary PCI for STEMI; 2013 ACCF/AHA Guideline for STEMI; 2013 ACC/AHA Guideline on Blood Cholesterol; 2017 ACC/AHA Focused Update on Non-Statin Therapies; 2018 ACC/AHA Guideline on Blood Cholesterol; 2017 AHA/ACC Guideline for Ventricular Arrhythmias and Sudden Cardiac Death; 2018 AHA Focused Update on ACLS Use of Antiarrhythmic Drugs; 2015 ACC/AHA Guideline for SVT; 2019 AHA/ACC Focused Update on Atrial Fibrillation; 2018 ACC/AHA Guideline on Bradycardia and Cardiac Conduction Delay; 2016 AHA/ACC Guideline on Lower Extremity PAD; ACCF/AHA 2009 Expert Consensus Document on Pulmonary Hypertension; CHEST 2014 Pharmacologic Therapy for Pulmonary Arterial Hypertension

Abbreviations: ACEi, ACE inhibitor; ACS, acute coronary syndrome; aPTT, activated prothrombin time; AS, aortic stenosis; BP, blood pressure; CABG, coronary artery bypass graft; CAD, coronary artery disease; CrCl, creatinine clearance; CVA, cerebrovascular accident; CVD, cardiovascular disease; DHA, docosahexaenoic acid; DM, diabetes mellitus; EPA, eicosapentaenoic acid; HTN, hypertension; INR, international normalized ratio; IU, international unit; IV, intravenous; kg, kilogram; mg, milligram; MI, myocardial infarction; ng, nanogram; PAD, peripheral arterial disease; PAH, pulmonary arterial hypertension; PCI, percutaneous coronary intervention; PDE-5, phosphodiesterase-5; PO, per os; RV, right ventricle; SC, subcutaneous; SSS, sick sinus syndrome; STEMI, ST-elevation myocardial infarction; SVT, supraventricular tachycardia; TIA, transient ischemic attack; wt, weight

Selected Reading

Al-Khatib SM, Stevenson WG, Ackerman MJ, et al. 2017 AHA/ACC/HRS Guideline for Management of Patients with Ventricular Arrhythmias and the Prevention of Sudden Cardiac Death: A Report of the American College of Cardiology Foundation / American Heart Association Task Force on Clinical Practice Guidelines and the Heart Rhythm Society. J Am Coll Cardiol, 2017.

American Heart Association. 2015 American Heart Association Guidelines Update for Cardiopulmonary Resuscitation and Emergency Cardiovascular Care. Circulation: 132 (18) supplement 2: S315–S573, 2015.

Amsterdam EA, Wenger NK, Brindis RG, et al. 2014 AHA/ACC Guideline for the Management of Patients with Non-ST-Elevation Acute Coronary Syndromes. A Report of the American College of Cardiology/American Heart Association Task Force on Practice Guidelines. J Am Coll Cardiol 130: e344–426, 2014.

Antman EM, Sabatine MS, Colucci WS, Gotto AM (eds). *Cardiovascular Therapeutics. A Companion to Braunwald's Heart Disease,* 4th ed. Philadelphia: Elsevier Saunders, 2013.

Arnett DK, Blumenthal RS, Albert MA, et al. 2019 ACC/AHA Guideline on the Primary Prevention of Cardiovascular Disease: A Report of the American College of Cardiology/American Heart Association Task Force on Clinical Practice Guidelines. J Am Coll Cardiol, 2019.

Carey RM, Calhoun DA, Bakris GL, et al. Resistant Hypertension: Detection, Evaluation, and Management: A Scientific Statement From the American Heart Association. Hypertension, 2018.

Chizner MA. *Clinical Cardiology Made Ridiculously Simple*. 5th ed. Miami, FL: Medmaster, Inc., 2019.

Chizner MA (ed). *Classic Teachings in Clinical Cardiology: A Tribute to W. Proctor Harvey, M.D.* Cedar Grove, NJ: Laennec Publishing Inc., 1996.

Dajani AS, Taubert KA, Wilson W, et al. Prevention of bacterial endocarditis: Recommendations by the American Heart Association. Circulation 96: 358–366, 1997.

Epocrates (Version 18.11) [Mobile application software]. Retrieved from http://itunes.apple.com.

Epstein AE, Dimarco JP, Ellenbogen KA, et al. ACC/AHA/HRS 2008 Guidelines for Device-Based Therapy of Cardiac Rhythm Abnormalities: A Report of the American College of Cardiology/American Heart Association Task Force on Practice Guidelines. J Am Coll Cardiol 51:2085–2105, 2008.

Executive Summary of the Third Report of the National Cholesterol Education Program (NCEP), Expert Panel on Detection, Evaluation, and Treatment of High Blood Cholesterol in Adults (Adult Treatment Panel III). JAMA 285 (19):2486–2497, 2001.

Fihn SD, Blankenship JC, Alexander KP, et al. 2014 ACC/AHA/AATS/PCNA/SCAI/STS Focused Update of the Guideline for the Diagnosis and Management of Patients With Stable Ischemic Heart Disease. A Report of the American College of Cardiology/American Heart Association Task Force on Practice Guidelines, and the American Association for Thoracic Surgery, Preventive Cardiovascular Nurses Association, Society for Cardiovascular Angiography and Interventions, and Society of Thoracic Surgeons. J Am Coll Cardiol; 64: 1929–1949, 2014.

Fihn SD, Gardin JM, Abrams J, et al. 2012 ACCF/AHA/ACP/AATS/PCNA/SCA/STS Guideline for the Diagnosis and Management of Patients with Stable Ischemic Heart Disease. A report of the American College of Cardiology Foundation/American Heart Association Task Force on Practice Guidelines, and the American College of Physicians, American Association for Thoracic Surgery, Preventive Cardiovascular Nurses Association, Society for Cardiovascular Angiography and Interventions, and Society of Thoracic Surgeons. Circulation; 126:3097–3137, 2012.

Fuster V, Harrington R, Narula J (eds). *Hurst's The Heart.* 14th ed. New York: McGraw-Hill, 2017.

Gerhard-Herman MD, Gornick HL, Barrett C, et al. 2016 AHA/ACC Guideline on the Management of Patients With Lower Extremity Peripheral Artery Disease: A Report of the American College of Cardiology/American Heart Association Task Force on Clinical Practice Guidelines. J Am Coll Cardiol, 2017.

Grundy SM, Stone NJ, Bailey AL, et al. 2018 ACC/AHA/AACVPR/AAPA/ABC/ACPM/ADA/AGS/APhA/ASPC/NLA/PCNA Guideline on the Management of Blood Cholesterol: A Report of the American College of Cardiology Foundation / American Heart Association Task Force on Clinical Practice Guidelines. J Am Coll Cardiol, 2018.

Hamilton RJ (ed). *Tarascon Pocket Pharmacopoeia*, 33rd ed. Burlington, MA: Jones & Bartlett Learning, 2019.

Hillis LD, Smith PK, Anderson JL, et al. 2011 ACCP/AHA Guideline for Coronary Artery Bypass Graft Surgery: A Report of the American College of Cardiology Foundation/American Heart Association Task Force on Practice Guidelines. Circulation 124:2610–2642, 2011.

Hirsch AT, Haskal ZJ, Hertzer NR, et al. ACC/AHA 2005 guidelines for the management of patients with peripheral arterial disease (lower extremity, renal, mesenteric, and abdominal aortic)—executive summary. J Am Coll Cardiol; 47(6):1239–1312, 2006.

James PA, Oparil S, Carter BL, et al. 2014 Evidence-Based Guidelines for the Management of High Blood Pressure in Adults. Report from the Panel

Members Appointed to the Eighth Joint National Committee, JNC 8. JAMA, 311(5):507–520, 2014.

January CT, Wann LS, Calkins H., et al., 2019 Focused Update of the 2014 AHA/ACC/HRS Guideline for the Management of Patients With Atrial Fibrillation: A Report of the American College of Cardiology/American Heart Association Task Force on Practice Guidelines and the Heart Rhythm Society: Executive Summary. J Am Coll Cardiol 2019.

Kusumoto FM, Schoenfeld MH, Barrett C, et al. 2018 ACC/AHA/HRS Guideline on the Evaluation and Management of Patients with Bradycardia and Cardiac Conduction Delay. A Report of the American College of Cardiology / American Heart Association Task Force on Clinical Practice Guidelines and the Heart Rhythm Society. J Am Coll Cardiol, 2018.

Levine GN, Bates ER, Blankenship JC, et al. 2011 ACCF/AHA/SCAI Guideline for Percutaneous Coronary Intervention: A Report of the American College of Cardiology Foundation/American Heart Association Task Force on Practice Guidelines/Society for Cardiovascular Angiography and Interventions. Circulation 124:2574–2609, 2011.

Moscucci M (ed). *Grossman and Baim's Cardiac Catheterization, Angiography and Intervention*. 8th ed. Philadelphia: Lippincott Williams & Wilkins, 2014.

Nishimura RA, Otto CM, Bonow RO, et al. 2014 AHA/ACC Guideline for the Management of Patients with Valvular Heart Disease: Executive Summary: A Report of the American College of Cardiology/American Heart Association Task Force on Practice Guidelines. J Am Coll Cardiol 63(22):2438–2488, 2014.

O'Gara PT, Kushner FG, Ascheim DD, et al. 2013 ACCF/AHA Guideline for the Management of ST Elevation Myocardial Infarction: Executive Summary: A Report of the American College of Cardiology Foundation/American Heart Association Task Force on Practice Guidelines. J Am Coll Cardiol: 61 (4): 485–510, 2013.

Opie LH, Gersh BJ (eds). *Drugs for the Heart*. 8th ed. Philadelphia: Elsevier Saunders, 2013.

Page RL, Joglar JA, Caldwell MA, et al. 2015 ACC/AHA/HRS Guideline for the Management of Adult Patients With Supraventricular Tachycardia A Report of the American College of Cardiology/American Heart Association Task Force on Clinical Practice Guidelines and the Heart Rhythm Society. J Am Coll Cardiol: 67 (13), 2016.

Panchal AR, Berg KM, Kudenchuk PJ, et al. 2018 American Heart Association Focused Update on Advanced Cardiovascular Life Support Use of Antiarrhythmic Drugs During and Immediately After Cardiac Arrest An Update to the American Heart Association Guidelines for Cardiopulmonary Resuscitation and Emergency Cardiovascular Care. Circulation. 2018.

Rosendorff C, Lackland DT, Allison M, et al. Treatment of Hypertension in Patients with Coronary Artery Disease, A Scientific Statement from the American Heart Association, American College of Cardiology, and American Society of Hypertension. J Am Coll Cardiol 65 (18): 1998–2038, 2015.

211

Patel MR, Calhoon JH, Dehmer GJ, et al. ACC/AATS/AHA/ASE/ASNC/ SCAI/SCCT/STS 2017 Appropriate Use Criteria for Coronary Revascularization in Patients With Stable Ischemic Heart Disease. A Report of the American College of Cardiology Appropriate Use Criteria Task Force, American Association for Thoracic Surgery, American Heart Association, American Society of Echocardiography, American Society of Nuclear Cardiology, Society for Cardiovascular Angiography and Interventions, Society of Cardiovascular Computed Tomography, and Society of Thoracic Surgeons. J Am Coll Cardiol, 2017.

Sabatine MS (ed). *Pocket Medicine*, 6th ed. Philadelphia, PA: Wolters Kluwer, 2017.

Seventh Report of the Joint National Committee on Prevention, Detection, Evaluation, and Treatment of High Blood Pressure. The JNC 7 Report. JAMA; 289 (19): 2560–2572, 2003.

Smith SC Jr., Benjamin EJ, Bonow RO, et al. AHA/ACCF Secondary Prevention and Risk Reduction Therapy for Patients with Coronary and Other Atherosclerotic Vascular Disease: 2011 Update. Circulation 124; 2458–2473, 2011.

Stone NJ, Robinson J, Lichtenstein AH, et al. 2013 ACC/AHA Guideline on the Treatment of Blood Cholesterol to Reduce Atherosclerotic Cardiovascular Risk in Adults. J Am Coll Cardiol 63(25):2889–2934, 2014.

Taichman DB, Ornelas J, Chung L, et al. Pharmacologic therapy for pulmonary arterial hypertension in adults: CHEST guideline and expert panel report. Chest, 2014.

Whelton PK, Carey RM, Aronow WS, et.al. 2017 ACC/AHA Guidelines for the Prevention, Detection, Evaluation, and Management of High Blood Pressure in Adults. A report of the American College of Cardiology/American Heart Association Task Force on Clinical Practice Guidelines. Hypertension, 2017.

Wilson W, Taubert KA, Gerwitz M, et al. Prevention of Infective Endocarditis. Guidelines from the American Heart Association. A Guideline from the American Heart Association Rheumatic Fever, Endocarditis, and Kawasaki Disease Committee, Council on Cardiovascular Disease in the Young, and the Council on Clinical Cardiology, Council on Cardiovascular Surgery and Anesthesia, and the quality of Care and Outcomes Research Interdisciplinary Working Group. Circulation 115: 2007.

Yancy C, Jessup M, Bozkurt B, et al. 2013 ACCF/AHA Guideline for the Management of Heart Failure. A Report of the American College of Cardiology Foundation/American Heart Association Task Force on Practice Guidelines. Circulation, 128: 1810–1852, 2013.

Zipes DP, Libby P, Bonow RO, Mann DL, Tomaselli GF (eds) *Braunwald's Heart Disease. A Textbook of Cardiovascular Medicine*. 11th ed. Philadelphia: Elsevier Inc., 2019.

Index

(bold numbers = key information)

A

Abciximab **36**, **181**
Accupril 94, 107, **187**
ACE inhibitors **19**, 110, **186**
Acebutolol **173**
Aceon **187**
Acetylsalicylic acid 32, **179**
ACLS algorithm **163**
Activase 38, **184**
Acute coronary syndrome (ACS) 61, 62, **70**
Acute heart failure 93, 100
Adalat 15, 99, **178**
Adcirca 156, **206**
Adempas 156, **208**
Adenocard 50, 58, 129, **193**
Adenosine **34**, 50, **58**, 81, 124, 129, **193**
ADP receptor antagonists 34, 70
Adrenalin **193**
Afeditab **178**
Aggrastat 36, 71, **181**
Aggrenox 34, **179**
Aldactone 31, 94, 99, **192**
Aldomet 106, **204**
Aldosterone antagonists 13, 31, 79, 94, 99, 107, 113, 134, **192**
Alirocumab 47, 73, 118, 122, **202**
Aliskiren 24, 107, 186, 189, **190**
Alpha-1 antagonists 12, **203**
Altace 20, 94, 99, 107, **187**
Alteplase **38**, 76, 89, 184
Amatine **193**
Ambrisentan 156, **206**

Amiodarone 5, 7, 26, 42, 50, **54**, 79, 95, 124, 131, 137, 173, 194, **200**
Amlodipine 15, 57, 65, **177**
Amrinone **28**
Anacin **179**
Angina 17, 32, 61, **64**
Angiomax 40, 71, **182**
Angioplasty 73, 84, 87
Angiotensin receptor antagonists **22**, **188**
Angiotensin receptor neprilysin inhibitor **23**, 94, **189**
Angiotensin-converting enzyme inhibitors **19**, **186**
Anistreplase **185**
Antara **201**
Antiarrhythmic agents **48**, **193**
Anticoagulants **38**, 40, 71, **182**
Antiplatelet agents **32**, 70, **179**
Aortic aneurysm **153**
Aortic dissection **152**
Aortic regurgitation **141**
Aortic stenosis **139**
Apixaban **40**, **182**
Apresoline 95, 96, 107, **204**
ARBs **22**, 73, **188**
Arixtra 40, 71, **183**
ARNI 23, **189**
Arrhythmias 48, **123**
Aspirin **32**, 68, 70, 87, 88, **179**
Atacand 22, 94, 107, **188**
Atenolol 12, 14, **54**, 65, 67, 99, 106, **173**
Atherosclerosis 44, 105
Atorvastatin 45, 117, **198**
Atrial fibrillation **123**

Coronary artery disease 61
Corvert 50, 56, 126, 196
Coumadin 32, 40, 72, 95, 126, 184
Coversyl 187
Cozaar 22, 94, 107, 188
CPR **161**, 163
Crestor 45, 73, 117, 199

D

Dabigatran **40**, 43, 126, 182, 195
Defibrillation 81, 82, 159, 160, 161
Demadex 30, 96, 100, 106
Digibind 26, 185
DigiFab 185
Digitalis 5, 7, 10, 16, 25-6, 29, 46, 53, **57**, 130-2, 137-8, 142, 162, 203
Digitek 185
Digoxin 6, 7, **25**, 31, 54, 57, 81, 82, 95, 99, 101, 123-134, 144, 156, 160, 173, 185
Digoxin immune fab 185
Dihydropyridine 15, 67, 99, 108, 113, 141, 177
Dilacor 15, 100, 107, 178
Dilated cardiomyopathy **134**
Diltiazem 7, 15, 50-52, **56**, 57, 65, 67, 69, 72, 79, 81, 83, 89, 90 99, 107, 113, 123, 130, 153, **178**, 196-200
Diovan 22, 94, 107, **189**
Dipyridamole 58, **179**, 193, 208
Direct renin inhibitor 19, **24**, 111, **190**
Direct thrombin inhibitors 33, 34, **39**, 40, 71, **182**
Direct vasodilators 107, **204**
Disopyramide 5, 49, **51**, 52, 126, 137, 138, 173, **194**
Diuretics **29**, 95, 106, **190**
Diuril 30, 95, 106, **191**
Dobutamine **26**, 84-87, 95, 97, 101, 156, **192**
Dobutrex 25, 95, 97, **192**
Dofetilide 50, **54**, 46, 126, 127, **195**
Dopamine **26**-28, 84-87, 95, 97, 101, **192**
Doxazosin 114, 107, 109, **203**

Dronedarone 50, **54**, 46, 95, **195**, 199, 200
Drug eluting stents 34, 35
Dynacirc 15, 99, 107, **177**
Dyslipidemia **115**

E

Ecotrin **179**
Edarbi 22, **188**
Edecrin 30, **190**
Edoxaban 34, **40**, 43, 126, **182**
Effient 35, 70, **180**
Eliquis 43, 126, **182**
Eminase **185**
Empagliflozin 63
Empirin **179**
Enalapril 20, 23, 94, 97, 99, 107, 110, **186**
Enalaprilat 110, **186**
Encainide **53**
Endothelin receptor antagonists **206**
Enoxaparin 33, 39, 41, 71, 76, 78, 87, 89, 90, **183**
Entresto 23, 94, 97, **189**
Epinephrine 12, **193**
EpiPen **193**
Eplerenone 13, 31, 87, 91, 94, 96, 114, **192**
Epoprostenol 156, **207**
Eprosartan 22, 94, 107, **188**
Eptifibatide 33, **36**, 68, 71, **181**
Esmolol 79, 81, 106, 110, 153, **174**
Ethacrynic acid 30, **190**
Evolocumab 47, 73, 118, 122, **202**
Ezetimibe 44, **47**, 73, 117, **203**

F

Factor Xa inhibitors 34, **39**, 40, 43, 68, 71
Felodipine 15, 16, 99, 107, **177**
Fenofibrate 46, 117, **201**
Fenofibric acid 46, 117, **201**
Fenoglide **201**
Fenoldopam 110, **204**
Fibrates 42, 44, 47, 117, 119, 198, **201**

217

Norpace 49, 52, 126, **194**
Norvasc 15, 69, 99, 107, zg
Novel oral anticoagulant (NOAC) 6, **40**, 43, 79, 126-7

O

Olmesartan 22, 94, **189**
Olmetec **189**
Omega fatty acids **202**
Omega-3-acid ethyl esters **202**
Opsumit 156, **206**
Orenitram **207**

P

P2Y12 inhibitor 68, 76, 88-9, 179
Pacemaker 81, 124-5, 132-3, 147-8, 150
Pacerone 126-7, **194**
PCSK-9 inhibitors **47**, 63, 68, 76, 88-9, **179**
Pentoxifylline **205**
Percutaneous coronary intervention (PCI) 6, 34-6, 39-41, 61, 63-4, 66, 68-71, 74-80, 86-94, 100, 150, 161-2, 179-84, 208
Pericarditis 75, 78, **88**, 95, 123-4, **157**-8
Perindopril **187**
Peripheral arterial disease 152, **154**, 208
Phenytoin **53**
Phenylephrine **193**
Phosphodiesterase inhibitors 26, **28**, 95
Pindolol 14, 173, **175**
Pitavastatin 45, 117, **199**
Plavix 6, 34, 70, 126, **179**
Plendil 15, 99, 107, **177**
Pletal 154, **179**
Potassium sparing diuretics 21, 30-**31**
Pradaxa 43, 126, **182**
Praluent 47, 73, 118, 122, **202**
Prasugrel **33-6**, 63, 68, 70, 76, 87-90, **180**
Pravachol 45, 117, **199**

Pravastatin 45, 117, **199**
Prazosin 107, **203**
Primacor 26, 28, 95, 97, **193**
Prinivil 20, 94, 99, 107, **187**
Prinzmetal's angina 14, 16-7, 61, 66-7
Procainamide 5, 49, **51**-52, 79, 81-5, 124-6, 130-1, 157, **197**
Procan 49, 52, 126, **197**
Procardia 15, 99, 107, 111, **178**
Pronestyl 52, 126, 131, **197**
Propafenone 7, 42, 49, **53**-4, 126-8, **197**
Propranolol 12, 13, **54**, 67, 99, 106, **175**
Prostanoids **207**
Pulmonary edema 30, 64, 85-6, 94, **100**-1, 109-10, 143
Pulmonary hypertension 16, 98, 143, 145-6, **155**-6, 205, 208
Pulseless electrical activity (PEA) 15, 18, 159, 160, 162-3, 165-6
Pulseless ventricular tachycardia 159, 163

Q

Questran 46, 117, 119, **200**
Quinaglute **198**
Quinapril 20, 94, 99, 107, **187**
Quinidex 49, **198**
Quinidine 5, 7, 26, 42, 49, **51**-2, 95, 197, **198**

R

Ramipril 20, 94, 99, 107, **187**
Ranexa 66, **177**
Ranolazine 66-7, **177**, 198, 200
Remodulin 156, **207**
Renin inhibitors 19, **24**, 107, 111
ReoPro 36, 71, **181**
Repatha 47, 73, 118, 122, **202**
Resistant hypertension **113**
Restrictive cardiomyopathy 94
Reteplase **38**, 71, 76, 78, 89, **185**
Revatio 156, **206**
Right ventricular infarction 84, **86**
Riociguat 156, 176, 206, **208**

RAPID LEARNING AND RETENTION THROUGH THE MEDMASTER SERIES:

CLINICAL NEUROANATOMY MADE RIDICULOUSLY SIMPLE, by S. Goldberg

CLINICAL BIOCHEMISTRY MADE RIDICULOUSLY SIMPLE, by S. Goldberg

CLINICAL ANATOMY MADE RIDICULOUSLY SIMPLE, by S. Goldberg and H. Ouellette

CLINICAL PHYSIOLOGY MADE RIDICULOUSLY SIMPLE, by S. Goldberg

CLINICAL MICROBIOLOGY MADE RIDICULOUSLY SIMPLE, by M. Gladwin, B. Trattler and C.S. Mahan

CLINICAL PHARMACOLOGY MADE RIDICULOUSLY SIMPLE, by J.M. Olson

OPHTHALMOLOGY MADE RIDICULOUSLY SIMPLE, by S. Goldberg

PSYCHIATRY MADE RIDICULOUSLY SIMPLE, by J. Nelson, W. Good and M. Ascher

CLINICAL PSYCHOPHARMACOLOGY MADE RIDICULOUSLY SIMPLE, by J. Preston and J. Johnson

USMLE STEP 1 MADE RIDICULOUSLY SIMPLE, by A. Carl

USMLE STEP 2 MADE RIDICULOUSLY SIMPLE, by A. Carl

USMLE STEP 3 MADE RIDICULOUSLY SIMPLE, by A. Carl

BEHAVIORAL MEDICINE MADE RIDICULOUSLY SIMPLE, by F. Seitz and J. Carr

ACID-BASE, FLUIDS, AND ELECTROLYTES MADE RIDICULOUSLY SIMPLE, by R. Preston

THE FOUR-MINUTE NEUROLOGIC EXAM, by S. Goldberg

MED SCHOOL MADE RIDICULOUSLY SIMPLE, by S. Goldberg

MEDICAL SPANISH MADE RIDICULOUSLY SIMPLE, by T. Espinoza-Abrams

MED'TOONS (260 humorous medical cartoons by the author) by S. Goldberg

CLINICAL RADIOLOGY MADE RIDICULOUSLY SIMPLE, by H. Ouellette and P. Tetreault

NCLEX-RN MADE RIDICULOUSLY SIMPLE, by A. Carl

THE PRACTITIONER'S POCKET PAL: ULTRA RAPID MEDICAL REFERENCE, by J. Hancock

ORGANIC CHEMISTRY MADE RIDICULOUSLY SIMPLE, by G.A. Davis

CLINICAL CARDIOLOGY MADE RIDICULOUSLY SIMPLE, by M.A. Chizner

CARDIAC DRUGS MADE RIDICULOUSLY SIMPLE, by M.A. Chizner and R.E. Chizner

ECG INTERPRETATION MADE RIDICULOUSLY SIMPLE, by M.A. Chizner

CARDIAC PHYSICAL EXAM MADE RIDICULOUSLY SIMPLE, by M.A. Chizner

PATHOLOGY MADE RIDICULOUSLY SIMPLE, by A. Zaher

CLINICAL PATHOPHYSIOLOGY MADE RIDICULOUSLY SIMPLE, by A. Berkowitz

ORTHOPEDICS MADE RIDICULOUSLY SIMPLE, by P. Tétreault and H. Ouellette

IMMUNOLOGY MADE RIDICULOUSLY SIMPLE, by M. Mahmoudi

CLINICAL BIOSTATISTICS AND EPIDEMIOLOGY MADE RIDICULOUSLY SIMPLE, by A. Weaver and S. Goldberg

ARE YOU AFRAID OF SNAKES?: A Doctor's Exploration of Alternative Medicine, by C.S. Mahan

ALLERGY AND ASTHMA MADE RIDICULOUSLY SIMPLE, by M. Mahmoudi

RHEUMATOLOGY MADE RIDICULOUSLY SIMPLE, A.J. Brown

THE STUTTERER'S APPRENTICE, by A. Splaver

CRITICAL CARE AND HOSPITALIST MEDICINE MADE RIDICULOUSLY SIMPLE, by M. Donahoe and M.T. Gladwin

CONSCIOUSNESS MADE RIDICULOUSLY SIMPLE: A Serious Resolution of the Mind/ Body Problem, by S. Goldberg

For further information, see http://www.medmaster.net or Email: info@medmaster.net.